THE
A 10 DAY QUICK WEIGHT LOSS & DETOX PLAN WITH A DIFFERENCE
DANIEL WAY TO WEIGHT LOSS

PHILIP BRIDGEMAN ND. BSC.

ANCIENT HEALTH & WEIGHT LOSS SECRETS REVEALED

Ark House Press
PO Box 1722, Port Orchard, WA 98366 USA
PO Box 1321, Mona Vale NSW 1660 Australia
PO Box 318 334, West Harbour, Auckland 0661 New Zealand
arkhousepress.com

GNB: Good News Bible
NASB: New American Standard Bible
NKJV: New King James Version
NIV: New International Version

All scriptural quotes unless marked with the above initials come from the Spirit
Filled Life Bible, New King James Version.

First published 2004 as 'Daniel's Diet'; due to its enormous success and
international release the book was upgraded and the name was changed in
2017 to 'Daniel's Way to Weight Loss'.
This book won third prize in the prestigious Living Now Book Awards (2011)
in the United States of America. It is also a best seller.

Cataloguing in Publication Data:
Bridgeman, Philip.
Daniels Way to Weight Loss - the 10-day detox & weight loss plan.
Includes index. ISBN 9780995421578
1. Bible. O.T. Daniel. 2. Reducing diets. 3.
Detoxification (Health). I. Title.

Design by initiateagency.com

A DIET PLAN THAT'S BEEN 'TESTED' SUCCESSFULLY FOR OVER 2000 YEARS AND WILL WORK FOR YOU TODAY!

'Please __Test me for 10 days on a diet of vegetables and water__'. (Daniel: 1 v 12)

"Please test your servants for 10 days, and let us be given some vegetables to eat and water to drink. Then let our appearance be observed in your presence, and the appearance of the youths who are eating the king's choice food: and deal with your servants according to what you see." (Daniel 1:12-13 NASB)

In Daniel 1:15-16 The Bible says, *"Well, at the end of the ten days, Daniel and his three friends looked healthier and better nourished than the youths who had been eating the food supplied by the king! So, after that the steward fed them only vegetables and water, without the rich foods and wines!"* (The Living Bible)

Daniel (around 605 BC), had just proven how powerful a 10-day vegetarian cleansing diet really was.

Achieve your ideal weight, regain your energy, live longer, look fantastic and learn to create yummy and healthy foods.

Ancient Wisdom combined with Modern Nutrition
This diet is based on the wisdom of 'Ancient Scriptures' and modern day nutrition. This diet bridges the gap between Bible times and Today and you can benefit from all that wisdom.

WELCOME TO 'DANIEL'S WAY' - TO WEIGHT LOSS

This Book and Diet Plan is based on both modern nutrition (from my 30 years in Clinical Practice) and Ancient Dietary Principles revealed in Daniel's Diet. This life changing healthy eating plan is found in the Ancient Scriptures of the Old Testament book of Daniel (Chapter 1).

This health plan and diet is a straight forward, short term program designed to help you lose weight, gently detox your body and regain your energy and improve your health. This diet bridges the gap between The Bible, Hippocrates (called the Father of Western Medicine) and now.

'I can confidently and unequivocally state that this diet plan works – WHY? Because of the thousands of success stories.'

The program is short term making the 10 day goal easy to commit to.

You will be eating 5 times a day, meaning no desperate hunger pains.

It is a gentle Detox, keeping in mind that toxicity is one driver of obesity. [1]

It is predominantly an alkaline diet (high acid levels are another factor in blocking weight loss).[2]

This diet is a Vegan Diet. Vegan means you eat NO animal product at all, including no eggs, milk and cheese.

It is also a Gluten Free diet.

Do you want to?

Lose weight

Regain energy

Remain healthy

Keep the weight off
Stop craving sugar/carbs
Break the cycle of illness
Overcome emotional eating
Make the most out of your life
Enhance your Spirituality by doing this partial 'Fast'

With so many products and weight loss systems in the market place how do you decide what is right for you? Nearly every person over 15 years old has tried a diet of some description, some people tell me "you name the diet and I've tried it, and I am still gaining weight?" I encourage you not to give up even if you have tried nearly every diet known to mankind. All you need is a plan that you can trust. My goal is to supply you with that plan.

Keep in mind that this Diet has the God factor added to it, and this makes all the difference.

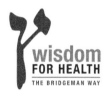

Email: philip@optusnet.com.au

DISCLAIMER:

This book is not intended to take the place of medical advice or treatment. Readers are advised to consult their own doctor regarding the treatment of their medical problems. People with serious health issues should be under professional supervision before attempting this diet. If you are taking any prescribed medication you should check with your doctor before using the recommendations in this book. This book is not meant to prescribe for any individual. All the names of individuals used as case histories have been changed. This book is based on the personal experience of the author. Neither the publisher, the author nor anyone involved in this books creation, takes any responsibility for possible consequences caused by any treatment, action or application of any herb, diet or preparation used by any person reading or following the information in this book.

To my Hero.

Alani Lily Maver my number 1 granddaughter. The most beautiful, sensitive and intelligent 'little fella' I have ever known. Who for the 8 months of her life showed me and everyone who had the privilege to meet her; what true courage is, and what life is really all about; family, love and life after death. Also to her mom Nova and dad Troy who are truly the best parents and I am so proud of them all.

AUTHOR'S INTRODUCTION...

In more than 20 years of treating overweight and sick people this diet is the single most effective tool I have ever used or witnessed. I have the testimonies to prove it. I have designed this book to teach and explain WHY you need to do the diet and change certain things in your lifestyle. By doing so - success is yours.

Our 21st century lifestyle has added many diseases to the world that are directly related to our modern day eating and drinking habits. Sad, but true! It makes sense, therefore, **that to overcome modern day diseases it is necessary to take some "modern" out of the equation and restore certain aspects of our lifestyles to how they were in previous times**. Not a step backwards but a restoration of what is good and beneficial in life.

This means getting back to the fundamentals of health and healing; fundamentals that The Bible teaches and those that Hippocrates, the recognized founder of modern medicine, recommended. Hippocrates also known for his profound quotes once said, *"Let food be your medicine and medicine your food."*

This is actually reiterating The Bible. *"…their fruit will be for food and their leaves for medicine."* (*Ezekiel 47:12*)

Daniel's Diet bridges the gap between The Bible, Hippocrates and Today. It teaches principles of health and healing that are necessary for our survival in this century. Keep in mind that a majority of the world's population is suffering some form of ill health and 70% or more of every illness is caused by what you do, or do not, put in your mouth. Daniel's Diet then gives you the opportunity to undertake a 10-day detox program, which is a practical answer to this modern era of ill health.

Over my years as a Naturopath and Nutritionist I have come to the following conclusion:

Firstly, the connection between your lifestyle and what you DO and DO NOT eat is of primary concern in the treatment and prevention of sickness and disease.

Secondly, the relationship between your environment and stress in relation to your health cannot be overlooked.

Thirdly, we must consider the human spiritual side in treatment of physical and emotional disharmony. If your physical body is sick and tired then it affects you spiritually and vice versa. You take your spirit with you wherever you go and in the condition that you are living at that time. Your mind, body and spirit are inseparable. Disease therefore is often a result of an imbalance between mind, body, and spirit. Try it for yourself, follow these guidelines and see the results.

**"Work with Jesus for your *Health* and *Healing*
– Not against Him"!**

Philip Bridgeman (BSc, N.D. Dip. Theo. Dip.Herb.Med)

CONTENTS

CONTENTS

CONTENTS

Part One

WISDOM FOR HEALTH

CHAPTER ONE

THE STORY OF DANIEL

I n Biblical history there was a man called Daniel. His inspiring life story is recorded in the Bible, in the book of Daniel, and this is where Daniel's Diet originated.

From Sunday school many may remember the story of Daniel and how he was thrown into the lion's den yet lived to tell the tale. But to me this wasn't Daniel's most heroic deed. I choose to remember him as the man who, under immense peer pressure and temptation from the finest foods and wines, ate a diet demonstrating a principle that we can all benefit from today.

History - Behind the Diet

Around 605 BC, Babylon's King Nebuchadnezzar, having conquered Jerusalem, ordered his aide to select from among the slaves, young men of Judah's royalty and nobility to attend Babylon's top University. Babylonians believed in integrating conquered people into their way of life and their intention here was to teach slave students the Chaldean language and literature so that they could be trained for important administration work within the government.

It was an intensive 3-year training program. All students lived on the palace grounds and were fed the finest meats, delicacies and wines from the king's own kitchen. There were no limits. Students were permitted to indulge in whatever they desired and to consume as much as they desired.

However, Daniel dared to be different. Wanting to be physical and spiritually healthy he chose not to eat these foods. I believe that the spiritual reasons behind the decision to not eat meat were due to the meat and some other foods probably being declared unclean by Moses law and therefore not 'kosher'. This would have been Daniels obvious priority but my emphasis is on the physical connection. Which is the overeating of rich food and wine affects your mental and physical health, proven in Daniel Ch 1 (and also modern nutritional science). So it's a fact that on the table Daniel shared with his three friends, fellow slaves, there was only a wide array of vegetables and clean water. When the Babylonian overseer heard that Daniel and his three friends, Shadrach, Meshach and Abednego, refused to eat the king's food he went and spoke with them.

Saying, *"The king has decided what you are to eat and drink, and if you don't look as fit as the other young men, he may kill you."* (GNB)

Daniel was so sure of his diet and of God's principles for health that he replied, *"Please test your servants for 10 days, and let us be given some vegetables to eat and water to drink. Then let our appearance be observed in your presence, and the appearance of the youths who are eating the king's choice food: and deal with your servants according to what you see."* (Daniel 1:12-13 NASB)

It is important to realize here that, since they were slaves, the stakes for Daniel and his friends were immense. If they were proven wrong, they would either be put to death or used as slave labor.

Proof That Daniel's Diet Works
The proof of this diet is declared in the Scriptures:

In Daniel 1:15-16 The Bible says, *"Well, at the end of the ten days, Daniel and his three friends looked healthier and better nourished than the youths who had been eating the food supplied by the king! So, after that the steward fed them only vegetables and water, without the rich foods and wines!"* (TLB)

Daniel had just proven how powerful a 10-day cleansing vegetarian diet really was.

Currently; I have literally thousands of successful (proven) testimonies to prove that this diet works extremely well (see more examples at the end of this book and on my face book page.) http://www.youtube.com/user/danielsdetox?feature=mhee

This is just three examples:

Dear Philip - I am writing to thank you for changing my life! I bought your book late last year wanting to "lose weight quickly before Christmas". I "did" the diet and lost quite a few centimetres and I have lost 11 pounds (5kg) all up and fit into all my old clothes. The great thing about your book is the advice and support throughout the book. It really helps to get to the end and beyond. **Jemma**

Dear Philip - I bought your book, Daniel's Way, and have gone on the diet three times, with great results each time. The last time I completed it I lost 11 pounds (5 kgs) and averaged about 1-2 inches (3-5cm) from hips, thighs, waist etc and I felt fantastic. **Kit.**

Dear Philip - I am very happy with my weight loss on your diet. I have lost at least 17 and half pounds (8 kilos) in 10 days on your diet plan. That's unprecedented!

My clothes are feeling looser and I am so excited because I now know I can live without soft drink, biscuits/slices/cakes and bread every day. **Belinda**

'How The Holy Spirit Revealed Daniel's Diet to Me?'

The awesome 'power of food' and what changing your eating habits can do for your physical, emotional and spiritual life, first came to my attention in the mid 1980's. I had graduated from Naturopathic College and just opened my first health clinic. At that time an epidemic of myalgic encephalomyelitis (ME); now known as chronic fatigue syndrome (CFS) or Adrenal fatigue — was spreading across Australia, Great Britain and the globe.

This 'mysterious' illness was causing much community concern for it was difficult to diagnose and was deemed incurable by most authorities. However, as it turned out, three diagnosed ME (chronic fatigue) sufferers came to consult with me in a two-week period and I soon discovered that with a determined lifestyle change, these 'so-called' incurable cases dramatically improved. The lifestyle changes included natural vitamin mineral and herbal supplements and a specific cleansing and rebuilding diet, **which this book is based on.**

Karen. D was one of these three sufferers who consulted with me and she happened to be the President of the Myalgic Encephalomyelitis Association for her region. Her progress in health was incredible, considering the terrible symptoms she had. Karen was so impressed with my treatment that she encouraged me to research this chronic fatigue problem and from that time on and for many years after I specialised in this area of health care. What frustrated me during my research was the lack of professional and medical data on this subject. In fact, I could find nothing specific on the topic. Most of the medical establishment didn't even recognise or believe the illness existed.

If the lack of information frustrated me as a researcher and practitioner, I knew just how discouraging it was to the actual CFS (ME) sufferers and their families. A majority of them had consulted with many doctors and specialists, most averaging twelve or more different practitioners before seeing me.

I was compelled to write a research paper that demonstrated that Chronic Fatigue Syndrome (CFS/ME) was a real and significant problem. I wished to inform people that there was help available to give them hope and a direction to follow. Understand that this was a very new and misunderstood phenomenon. The research paper I presented was basically ignored by the mainstream system, so to get the information to as many people as possible, I self-published a book called *There is a Cure for Chronic Tiredness – ME*. This book did help many people at that time and my work in this field led to me being nominated for the **Australian Bicentennial Awards for the Pursuit of Excellence.**

After treating many people with ME (CFS) and various other illnesses I began to realise that there was a missing link in the overall recovery of some patients. I was treating people with natural remedies with success, but what about the 'spiritual' side of the holistic approach to healing? We are tri-part beings—soul, body and spirit—and so must look after each part or we have an imbalance that can only lead to ill health in one or more parts.

Then I discovered a diet that was 2500 years old.

At this time I felt a calling to attend Bible College and so I closed my clinic and committed to 3 years full time at Rhema Bible College Perth.

Daniel's Diet was revealed to me:
It is amazing that half way through my third year at Bible College, God revealed to me a diet principle in the Bible that was a specific weight loss, detoxification and rejuvenation diet. It was nearly identical to the one I had been using in my clinic previously, **but the big difference was that here was a specific diet based on the Word of God.** This distinction was one that joined the spiritual link to natural healing principles.

*God actually spoke very clearly to me while I was reading Daniel Chapter One; He said that this diet is the **'Way'** to teach people to receive health and healing. That I was already knowledgeable on the system of nutrition but now use this plan based on Daniel's Diet and to go teach it and 'prove it to be so. This profound revelation changed my life forever and I remember it as clear as if it was yesterday. I was so impacted that I went immediately to my senior pastor and told him the story and he confirmed my idea and so I left college that very day and started to implement this teaching into a healing ministry. Within weeks I had a bona fida weekly healing ministry in action inside my church. The anointing was so strong people came from many other churches to my meetings. The anointing continued as within just a few months of hearing from God I was promoted to leading the Rhema Church Healing Ministry as well as my own. Then, before the year was finished I was asked to become a teacher in the Bible College and I was soon teaching my previous class mates, which could only be called a 'God' promotion. The next logical step was to write a book and so the original Dan-*

iel's Diet was written and now rewritten to become 'Daniel's Way to Weight Loss'.

I was tested on this Diet - just as Daniel was tested!

Again and again it has passed the test!

Since 1995 Daniel's Diet has been put through many public tests, from whole church congregations, individual and families plus live on radio (Sonshine FM. 98.5 in Perth, Western Australia). This is the radio station I has a weekly health segment on and they decided to 'test', or trial the 10-day diet plan on air with six of their announcers and staff. They were all weighed and measured before commencing the Daniel's Diet for 10 days. After the 10 days I had every one weigh in and measure again; the results were fantastic.

Everyone lost weight (from 4 -7 kg) and felt healthier, more clear-headed, less tired and more energetic than before. Some more compelling results included a staff member who had chronic pain in her feet due to calcium 'spurs'. She had to wear special shoes with in-built soles and could not walk without debilitating pain—she was healed of all pain and discomfort, in just 10 days. Also two radio announcers were diabetics; their blood sugar readings reduced from 14 and 15 to the healthy level of 5 (this took a few weeks longer and with the help of specific herbs I prescribed for them because of their special condition – more on diabetes later in this book).

In more than 20 years of treating overweight and sick people, this diet is the single most effective tool I have ever used or witnessed.

While I was having moderate success before, helping people individually, now I witness it multiplying to whole church congregations and the many testimonies I receive via email etc. I am witnessing today in my ministry many thousands of people who are being healed and set free of problems found in their bodies, souls and spirit.

Summary:

God has shown me that He has a health plan for us, but it is apparent that not many people know this plan. Therefore, it's not a new concept, confirmed to me when a local pastor said to me after I taught at his church in the south of Western Australia, ' This message is one of restoration, which means restoring or returning to God's best for us.'

This takes us back to the beginning—Genesis 1-29: *And God said, "See, I have given you every herb that yields seed which is on the face of all the earth, and every tree whose fruit yields seed; to you it shall be for food."*

CHAPTER TWO

A HEALTH PLAN FOR EVERY BODY

Daniel's Diet is for everybody - young, old, thin, over-weight, fit or unfit. This diet is so good that every person who tries it will be rewarded by varying degrees of good health, weight loss, clarity of mind and improved energy and vitality.

Mention the word diet to many people and immediately it conjures up thoughts of going hungry, not enjoying meals, weighing and measuring foods or surviving only on lettuce. Yet in reality diet means our manner of living and our current eating habits. It's not about starving and missing out, but about self-control and choosing how to eat and live.

In these days of quick fix solutions, which include take-away or fast foods, it is important to consider that the fastest option is not always the most beneficial. This is why, when trying to improve our health and weight it is also important to examine our entire lifestyle not just the food. A diet should not limit us to unexciting meals or require long hours without eating. It should allow us to eat 3-5 times a day with the only restrictions being on harmful and non-essential foods.

Picture the person you want to be - healthy, energetic, vibrant and happy; then read on because I believe you can achieve your ideal goals and image. Everyone can. I believe there is always an answer to any dietary or health problem or situation. I see Daniel's Diet as being this answer. .

Daniel's Diet is, in my experience, one of the most profound, life changing and healthiest diets I have seen in my 25 years as a health practitioner. But don't take my word for it, I also have countless testimonies from everyday people that have tried the diet and love the results.

I challenge you to take the step of faith and see what Daniel's Diet will do for you!

I'm sure that if most people realized exactly what they were doing to their bodies by consuming processed, pre-packaged and fast foods, they would make a life changing decision away from it and never look back. After all, no person in his or her right mind would choose to feed themselves, or their family, slow acting poisons. Yet, this is what most people are doing on a daily basis by eating these products.

Food manufacturers know that adding sugars (such as High Fructose Corn Syrup), salt, chemicals, animal fat and taste enhancers (such as mono sodium glutamate - MSG) to products can pervert the consumers' taste buds. This perversion leaves us craving any pre-chosen flavor, often to the point of addiction. It's a sober thought that we and our children can be pre-programmed, through our taste buds to eat food that is harmful to us. They also know that using this knowledge can be money in the bank for them. After all, any product that customers just 'have to have' will sell itself. I'm sorry to be the one to pass on the news but the consumer's health and well-being is neither the motivation nor the priority of manufacturers who use this information to their advantage, but it must become yours.

"There is a way that seems right to a man but its end is the way of death." (Proverbs 14:12).

This is in part why I wrote Daniel's Way to Weight Loss; to provide information on why we should change our eating habits. To explain how everyone can start the process of detoxifying their body and overcoming the cravings for these harmful and addictive foods. Also to explain why change is necessary and the dangers we all face by following modern diets. If you understand the why and how then you can make your own choices and do something about your health situation - wisdom and knowledge stimulate change, which brings success.

But besides that, Daniel's Diet is such a successful diet it demanded to be written for everyone not just my patients and church. By understanding, and following this diet's basic principles for 10 days it's possible to start regaining control over your body's health and weight. Starting from today your taste buds can slowly revert back to their original state, leaving you free to enjoy salads, vegetables and fruit more than ever.

Detoxifying and overcoming cravings is a vital step in the path back to good health.

This health plan enables you to have the freedom to choose what foods you want to eat and not be under the control of others. Following any restricted diet for a week or two will help a person lose weight - but what about after the diet? Will the weight come back? Will the old eating patterns return? This book is the beginning of the journey towards health and understanding. It's designed to give answers, advice, direction and wisdom - not just for the short term, but for the long term too. However, all journeys must commence with the first important step – you must choose to follow in Daniel's footsteps.

Is Your Diet and Lifestyle Harming You?

It's staggering to consider that what we do, or don't, put into our mouths causes at least 70% of all our disease and ill health.

In America, Australia and New Zealand (the statistics are very much the same - we are vying for first place as the 'fattest nations on earth', a staggering 61% are either overweight or obese. Even more concerning is the high ratio of overweight children in our society.

Weight loss is a vitally important subject and not just a cosmetic issue. It is so important for self-image, self-esteem. However it goes way beyond that – why? Because since 2012, the contribution of obesity to ill health is now greater than that of tobacco smoking [1]. Obesity is a major driver in many health problems people face. Fat reduction has been demonstrated to reduce the risk of developing these chronic diseases.

The media regularly reports that diabetes in our general population is reaching epidemic proportions, to say nothing of the many sicknesses that relate to self-abuse. In other words we are harming ourselves through our eating and lifestyle.

Ailments that include:

Strokes	Chronic tiredness
Heart problems	Low energy/Tired all the time
Hypoglycaemia	Depression (some)
Metabolic Syndrome	Poor concentration/memory
Headaches	ADHD (Attention Deficit Hyperactive Disorders)
High/low blood pressure	Cancer's (some)
Hormone issues	Arthritis
Skin problems	High cholesterol
Overweight/Obesity	

These figures alone should be enough to emphasize the need for an easy to follow, successful and healthy cleansing diet like the Daniel's Diet. Yet, the above is hardly surprising when we discover the most common items purchased in our supermarkets.

Best Sellers in Australian Supermarkets [2]
1. Coca-Cola, 375ml
2. Coca-Cola, 1L
3. Coca-Cola, 2L
4. Diet Coke, 375ml
5. Cherry Ripe chocolate
6. Nestlé's condensed milk
7. Tally Ho cigarette papers
8. Mars Bar chocolate
9. Kit-Kat chocolate
10. Crunchie chocolate Bar
11. Eta 5-star margarine, salt reduced
12. Heinz Baked Beans
13. Double-Circle tinned beetroot
14. Diet Coke, 1L
15. Bushell's tea

16.   Cadbury Dairy Milk Chocolate
17.   Pepsi Cola, 375ml
18.   Coca-Cola, 1.5L
19.   Kellogg's Cornflakes
20.   Maggie 2-minute chicken noodles
21.   Generic brand lemon drinks
22.   Panadol tablets, 24 pack

Fruit: The Undervalued Food

A classic example of our misaligned food intake concerns fruit. It's the least eaten of the five main food groups, yet it should be the greatest. We probably all know that, but we are still not consuming enough.

In a recent nutritional survey people were asked what they had eaten the day before:

90% of people had eaten cereals, cereal products, coffee, bread, milk, and milk products. (You will understand the full significance of this as you read though the book.)

Over half the people had eaten no fruit at all. In fact a CSIRO report in Australia showed that just one percent of people avoided junk food and the dietary habits of over 86500 adults over 12 months and four out of five people had a below - par diet [3].

Yet, even more concerning; 90% of the people saw no need to change their eating habits. They either falsely thought they were eating healthy or did not relate sickness to their lifestyle.

I am sorry but you do have to change if you want good health, weight loss and longevity of life.

God has given us food to eat and enjoy. In fact food and water are our only source of energy. So we have been designed to enjoy and desire food to ensure that we do eat regularly, this way we do not miss out on the life giving qualities that are found in our natural foods.

Gods plan is that we eat more foods from Gods Garden, food that is full of life and healing potential and NOT so much manmade and adulterated foods which are void of life and actually will cause you harm, in the short and long term consumption.

Because of so many easily accessible modern day foods, we are constantly faced with choices and temptations. Every day we have to choose which food we eat, I want to help you decide correctly. WHY? Because there is a sowing and reaping principle in life and we will reap the consequences of those decisions. My desire is that you reap good health and longevity of life, and this book and my teaching is the foundation you can now build on, to live that long and healthy life.

Snack Statistics in America [4]

Snack time presents an excellent opportunity to substitute fruits and vegetables for less healthy options. However; The National Health and Nutrition Examination Survey (NHANES III, a federally sponsored survey) analysis showed the most frequently reported foods eaten at snack time for American elementary school-age children are, in order:

1. Soft drinks (the number one source of calories in the United States)
2. Salty snacks such as potato chips, corn chips and popcorn
3. Cookies
4. Non-chocolate candy
5. Artificially flavored fruit beverages
6. Whole milk and chocolate milk
7. Two percent/reduced fat milk
8. White bread
9. Chocolate candy
10. Cake
11. Ice cream

This kind of thinking and resultant eating habits are against God's health principles; and the dietary guidelines recommended by USA and Australian health authorities.

When faced with reports like this it's no mystery to me why there are epidemics of obesity, diabetes, Chronic Fatigue Syndrome, heart problems, arthritis, depression, Attention Deficit Hyperactive Disorders

(ADHD) and cancer, etc.

After many years of clinical evidence in individual diet analysis I see that numerous people think they are eating a good diet, but in fact they are not. Many others know that certain foods are good or bad for them yet using that knowledge to their advantage is another thing.

The question that begs to be asked is – WHY?

Why do people on an ever-increasing scale eat food that is making them?

- Sick?
- Tired?
- Overweight?
- Depressed?
- Age prematurely, with a poor quality of life?

The answer to this question is complex and the causes involve mind, body and spirit issues. That is why during this book I discuss not only food habits but also the connection between physical, spiritual, mental and emotional health. Just following a diet is not always the complete answer.

Over 80% of the population suffers, in varying degrees, from sickness and tiredness.

Many think of this as normal, putting up with headaches, menstrual discomfort or pain, arthritis, general pain, gut discomfort, obesity, tiredness, loss of libido, infertility etc. The current health of our nations demonstrates to me just how important the content of this book is for everyone, but especially for parents and guardians. If children are exposed to good eating habits during the early stages of their lives, their chances of remaining healthy in adult years is dramatically increased. And again I'm talking here of good health in body, mind and spirit, not just the physical. The Bible says to train your children in the way they should go, (Proverbs. 22:6) this not only means spiritual matters but also practical and dietary matters.

We only have to look at the overcrowded hospital situation to see how bad the health of our nation has become and how urgent it is that we find a solution.

Why Do We Get Sick?

Do you ever stop and ask WHY?

- "Why have I got this symptom?"
- "Why do I keep getting sick?"
- "What is causing my pain?"
- "Why can't I lose weight?"
- "Why can't I maintain any weight loss?"
- "Why am I always tired or feeling generally 'Yuck'?"

The next question I encourage you to ask yourself and God is, "What can I do to fix the problem and to change the situation?"

Pain, tiredness, sickness, obesity and depression are all warning signs.

Once any of the warning signs are felt, surely the question needs to be asked – what is going on here and why? Pain and discomfort in this context are our best friends; they are our body's way of alerting us to problems. But we need to treat the warning sign correctly, not just cover the symptom with a quick fix.

Remember that pain is a guide; a guide to seeking the reason or cause and a warning that to prevent further problems we need to do something about it. It may take professional help to identify some of the symptoms of sicknesses, like high blood pressure, thyroid malfunction, cancer, depression, and arthritis, etc. But once the diagnosis is made, what is the next step?

Do you feel encouraged to accept a quick fix solution i.e. taking painkillers or antibiotics to overcome the problem? If so, this can often be no more help than putting a band-aid over the symptom. It covers the immediate pain or discomfort but a far more wise action would be to treat the cause.

Taking drugs for extended periods of time will not fix this scenario and in many cases will only make the situation worse. The quicker the warning signs are listened to, the easier it is to prevent the problem developing.

Diet and lifestyle are often the reasons why people get sick. What is necessary to correct this situation should now be obvious – a change in diet and lifestyle and the use of natural remedies where at all possible. Obviously in many advanced situations medication is necessary to keep a person alive and you should never stop taking them, but even so a change of diet is necessary for long-term health.

It is, by Gods design, that our bodies get all the necessary energy for life and healing from the ingredients contained in natural foods.

Take control of your own health. Remember approximately 70% of all ill health comes from what people are putting, or not putting, in their mouths.

Please note: There is always a place for drug therapy. NEVER go off prescribed medication without your doctor's consent. However, if you make lifestyle changes and want to use natural therapies, work towards lowering your medication until the time when it is safe to come off it – with the help and timing of your doctor.

Proven Benefits of Daniel's Diet (Daniel's Way)
(Taken from actual case histories)
After years of treating numerous people of all ages and from varied backgrounds, with nearly any disease you care to mention, I have learned one undeniable fact.

By initially concentrating on improving a person's physical, spiritual and emotional health, beneficial side effects occur automatically. Side effects such as; weight loss, tiredness, lethargy and the disappearance of many other negative symptoms of ill health.

The proven benefits include:
- Body - detoxified
- Bloating (intestinal) - gone

- Blood Pressure - improved
- Concentration - enhanced
- Cholesterol – lowered
- Cravings (sugar, refined carbohydrates & savory) - overcome
- Depression - lessened – mood improved
- Diabetes - improved
- Energy level – higher
- Excessive night-time urination - disappeared
- Fertility - increased
- Fluid retention – gone
- Food allergies and addictions - recognized and overcome
- Good health - renewed and maintained
- Hair and nail strength - improved
- Headaches - disappeared
- Hot flushes - disappeared
- Hypoglycemia - improved
- Immunity to recurring illness - strengthened
- Insomnia - disappeared
- Irritable Bowel Syndrome and stomach complaints -disappeared
- Menstrual problems and PMS - disappeared
- Mind - clearer and sharper
- Negative health symptoms - reversed
- Organs and tissues - stimulated into proper function
- Overeating - overcome
- Recovery from illness and drug treatments - assisted
- Reflux and indigestion - disappeared
- Skin problems (eczema, acne and dermatitis) - improved
- Spirituality - enhanced
- Stamina - increased
- Sugar cravings - overcome
- Tiredness – disappeared
- Self-Image improved
- Weight loss – accomplished

CHAPTER THREE

TOXIC, WHO ME?

Whether we are aware of it or not, virtually, everyone today is re-acting to stress, and polluted, degraded food, air and water. As a result, many of us have developed or will develop some form of health complaint.

Sadly, this ill health is often the consequence of our own actions. A consequence that I am sure was not in the original plan for us.

Jesus said, "*...I have come in order that you might have life - life in all its fullness.*" (John 10.10 TEV)

It is, however, up to us to individually make the choice to secure this fullness and better health for the future.

We need to adopt an attitude that says:
- "I want to be a good steward (caretaker) of my body"
- "I can do something about my health."
- "I want to and will change."
- "I won't become another medical statistic."
- "I will take back control."
- "I am in control of my lifestyle."

Toxins from the following have a detrimental effect on us:

• Polluted air and water	• Chemicals	• Caffeine
• Allergies	• Stress	• Alcohol
• Legal and illegal drugs	• Cigarettes	• Sugar

• Negative emotions (which there are many; e.g. Resentment, anger, unforgiveness, unfulfilled desires, bitterness, fear, self hatred, regrets, etc). Some people may be surprised that stress and negative emotions release harmful toxins inside our body. It does!

And if coming to terms with the toxic food additives isn't hard enough, pesticide and chemical residues poison much of the food we consume today before it even reaches the supermarket shelves.

Throughout the relay of supply and demand - from grower/manufacturer to wholesaler to retailer - foods are stored, frozen, refined, incorrectly cooked, added to and subtracted from, until they finally reach the consumer often containing absolutely no nutritional benefit at all.

In the case of some packet cereals and ready-cooked fast food, the packaging is more nutritious than the contents! And when it comes to many of the breakfast cereals filling tables across the world, people might believe they are getting a healthy start to the day but in actual fact their bowl might just as well be filled with gooey sugar laden sweets.

The sad truth is that most people are eating unhealthy foods with a frequency that is well beyond the amount that their body can healthily cope with.

From my experience the average person's diet comprises of at least 75% non-essential food.

This is a frightening figure when you consider it only takes approximately 25% of non-essential food to cause health problems.

Poor diet is often overlooked as the reason for health problems because a lot of symptoms are delayed ten to twenty years so they are often blamed on something else.

Depression and anxiety, caused through chemical imbalances within the brain, may also be attributed to diet. Our brain operates on pure fuel, if it's fed dirty fuel it will malfunction.

If you are still not convinced of the need to detoxify, try completing the following questionnaire.

Do I Need To Detoxify? Questionnaire
Please tick the questions that you answer YES.
- Do you experience stress regularly?

- Do you get fewer than seven hours of sleep every night?
- Do you wake most mornings feeling tired, lethargic
- Do you regularly feel tired, apathetic or lack energy?
- Do you eat less than 3 different fruits a day?
- Do you eat a salad/raw vegetable meal every day?
- Do you overeat?
- Do you eat processed or take away foods, more than once per week?
- Do you often find yourself craving for sweet or savory foods?
- Do you exercise, less than thirty minutes every second day?
- Are you overweight?
- Do you suffer from a recurring illness?
- Do you suffer from stomach pains, heartburn, indigestion, excess wind (gas) or a bloated stomach?
- Are you constipated?
- Are you a cancer patient?
- Do you have high blood pressure or high cholesterol?
- Do you experience cold hands and/or feet regularly?
- Do you have a history of antibiotic use?
- Do you suffer from allergies or hay fever/sinus?
- Do you get canker sores or ulcers in your mouth or on your lips?
- Do you suffer from headaches?
- Do you notice a lack of concentration, loss of memory or perhaps mental 'fog' (cognitive impairment)?
- Do you suffer from depression, anxiety or nervousness, or mood swings?
- Do you suffer from arthritis, joint pain or stiffness?
- Do you have any kind of skin problems, including skin cancer?
- Do you have blurred vision?
- Do you suffer from red or sore eyes?
- Do you have dark circles under your eyes?

WOMEN ONLY
- Do you experience irregular cycles or excessive menstrual flow?
- Do you experience any PMS, e.g. depression, crying too easily, or moodiness around your period time?
- Do you experience cramps, pain or bloating?
- Do you experience uncomfortable or distressing menopausal symptoms?

To have more than TWO of these symptoms indicates a toxic build up. Therefore, anyone who answered YES to two or more questions would benefit greatly from following Daniel's Diet.

What Happens When A Body Has Toxic Overload?
Each of us was uniquely designed and we are all incredible and beautiful creations. Every one of us deserves to be healthy enabling us to enjoy life and fulfill the potential and destiny that each of us was born for.

Given the right opportunities our minds and bodies are all self-repairing.
Through a good diet, a healthy lifestyle, adequate sleep, relaxation, and positive thinking, we will generate an abundance of physical energy and brainpower sufficient for any task, including healing and longevity.

However, this result is only accomplished by always taking care of the mind, body and spirit and feeding them the right ingredients. If these steps aren't taken then unfortunately our bodies will have lower thresholds of energy and immunity when it comes to preventing disease and living a normal, healthy life.

The human body is designed to cleanse and eliminate toxins automatically. But sadly, in current times it generally can't keep pace with the quantity of contaminants coming through. The toxins (by-products of chemicals, poisons and foreign substances) that we knowingly or unknowingly put into our bodies gradually build up to a level beyond what we can naturally eliminate on a daily basis.

When these levels get too high, our bodies, recognizing toxins as foreign substances and being unsure of the best way to handle them, store them in our fat cells - its last line of protection. This is, in part, how cellulite is formed along with dimples on thighs and the common 'potbelly'. The fat around the waist is the most dangerous. Fat around the waist means fat around the heart. Diabetes risk increases with waist measurement. Subcutaneous fat around the hips is not as dangerous, so if you have fat around the hips or 'rear end' it means your body is protecting your heart and storing the fat in this area and it's better than around your heart. This continuous accumulation of multi-mixtures of toxins sticks to arteries and veins, where it aggravates the tissue, causing inflammation, hardened arteries and interferes with the stomach. Our elimination or filter systems and organs, the liver, kidneys and skin, are the next to be overloaded. Skin problems may occur at this stage, along with puffy and dark circles under the eyes.

Hair and nails can lose their luster and develop other problems. The final result is an overall unhealthy appearance of the person that we each could and should be, leaving us thinking, "whatever happened to that lovely and vital person I was predestined to be?"

In the final analysis, our health depends upon the circulation of pure blood. The composition of our blood depends mainly upon the food we eat and the water we drink.

If the right foods are eaten, clean blood is generated and the liver, kidney, heart, brain and all other organs function normally.

Sadly, the ideal is becoming less common and harder to achieve. But it's worth remembering that under ideal conditions disease is practically impossible. Interestingly, according to the Bible during the Exodus when the Israelites were brought out of Egypt and trekked across the Wilderness none of them got sick. Why? Because they were in an ideal environment, plenty of clean water, clean air, exercise, a healthy restricted diet and a powerful spiritual connection. Their body, mind and spirit were in harmony and this is the key to a long and healthy life.

Eliminating the Poisons

By **detoxifying regularly** everyone can assist their bodies to regenerate and self repair, just like it's been designed to do. I often say at my Church talks, "Work with Jesus for your healing – not against Him".

Detoxification is simply, 'getting rid of any harmful and foreign substances from the body.' Detoxification is important because it helps us withstand the daily bombardment of free radicals (toxins) on our mind and body.

Without doubt prevention is better than cure. Ironically, prevention is also the simplest solution and yet the least practiced. By regularly detoxing there is less likelihood of experiencing the unfavorable side effects and illnesses of a modern day lifestyle.

When a person becomes sick, they should undertake a regimented detoxification process, like Daniel's Diet. The sicker people are, the more necessary the need to take supplements and the stricter and harder the detoxification should have to be. Therefore, it makes sense to undergo this detox process on a regular basis, to maintain a healthy system and to avoid serious illness.

A Good example is Karen. M - (Age late 20's), when she was told she was going to die by the doctors. Why because she was obese and to the point she was in hospital because of the resultant health problems she developed. This is her email to me: '*Thanks Philip - This Diet plan not only changed my life but probably saved it. I was obese, had very low self image, and in hospital the doctors were worried for my immediate health. Now things are so different; I have followed your 10 day diet three times in the last 2 months, (In between the 10 days I have followed your 'The 6 week Low Carb' diet.) Praise God, I lost 22 lbs or 10 Kilos every time I did the 10 days (66 lbs or 30 kg in total). I am now out of the danger zone and no longer need to go to the hospital. My confidence is returning and I have so much more energy, sleeping much better at night (had sleep apnoea). Thank you for your part in my way to good health, better self-esteem and a more vital life - Karen M.'* Karen is fully committed to good health choices now and has become a good friend of mine since this time and has appeared on radio with me giving her testimony and is part of my ministry team. See the progression of Karen's testimony on my YouTube interview – see link above.

CHAPTER FOUR

HOW TO LESSEN THE TOXIC OVERLOAD

Our bodies are designed to be extremely tough and resilient to a lot of abuse. They are self-cleansing, self-regenerating and self-repairing, given the right conditions and we have all been given a wonderful immune system as well, but there are limits.

The reason most of us are not as well as we would like to be is because our bodies are battling to clear themselves of the overburden of toxic waste and other rubbish from our diet and environment.

The Bible calls every human body, 'The Temple of The Holy Spirit'. Indicating just how important each one of us is and how vital it is that we look after our bodies. Our body is, after all, the only one we get and if it's the home of the Holy Spirit, then we had better look after it.

It only takes a little effort to lighten the overload of toxins and the rewards are truly wonderful.

So let's identify some common everyday culprits and start cutting the daily hit list back to a manageable quota.

Diet	Drugs (legal and illegal)	Alcohol
Petro chemicals	Exhaust fumes	Pesticides/herbicides
Cigarettes	Chemotherapy	Radiation
Stress	Carpet dust and house moulds	Sugar/table salt
Tap water	Cosmetics	Aerosol sprays

The complete list of items causing toxins within our society is long and if studied can be alarming. However, there are lots of practical and simple ways to shorten the list and thereby, take some pressure off our bodies.

I suggest correcting as many of the following list as possible.

- Use natural toothpaste – containing no Sodium Lauryl Sulphate or Sodium Laureth Sulphate.
- Change toothbrushes approximately every one - two months and apply one or two drops of 100% tea tree oil to the brush (once/twice week) to help eliminate germs.(If you have allergy to tea tree do not use it.)
- Avoid lead/mercury teeth fillings. Request teeth are refilled with white or gold fillings.
- Lipsticks, cosmetics, soaps and body lotions should be chemical free. This includes sun block lotions.
- Avoid deodorants that contain chemicals and aluminum (most do).
- Use shampoos (or any cosmetic) that contain no Sodium Lauryl Sulphate.
- Use natural hair dyes.
- Use a dry skin brush on your body daily (natural bristles only).
- Use unbleached and non-perfumed toilet paper.
- Wear only cotton or woolen underwear.
- Wash clothes and dishes in a natural or low allergy detergent, then rinse well.
- Use water filters on drinking water and showerheads.
- Avoid using a microwave to heat or prepare food.
- Avoid eating fast/take away foods as much as possible.
- Don't drink out of plastic or synthetic cups. Baby's bottles should be glass.
- Use less soft plastics for food storage and throw out aluminum cookware.
- Avoid living near major power lines & phone towers.

- Minimize mobile phone usage and use radiation protectors on the phone.
- Use a radiation shield over your computer screen.
- Have wooden or tile floors to cut down on house dust/mite pollutants.
- Always keep a window open to let in the fresh air, (if safe).
- Eat organic food where possible.

Stress

Stress reactions inside our body cause the release of certain oxidants (toxins) into our blood. It also depletes our bodies of nutrients. These factors are common to everyone because we live in a society that has stress built into its very framework. If these stress levels grow too high and are not addressed as they appear, eventually they will lead to sickness and disease.

It's possible for every person to manage their stress levels by including regular periods of rest, sleep, holidays and relaxation in their life. Moderate, regular exercise is a great way of de-stressing the body. Meditation and prayer, laughing, healthy sex in marriage and enjoying life are also 'Stress Busters'. Doing these things releases natural neurochemicals (endorphins) into our brain, making us feel good and happy.

Antioxidants are also very helpful in combating toxins released by stress. And, once again, adopting a preventative approach is the best policy.

Stress drains the body of:
- Vitamin C
- B Vitamins (multi)
- Magnesium
- Minerals (multi electrolytes)

An explosive argument or making pressing business or social decisions can drain huge quantities of these nutrients out of our system in just minutes, quickly depleting our body's reserves. This is especially true of the B and C vitamins, which are not stored in the body and need to be replaced daily through diet. In the food charts included in this book you will notice B and C vitamins are in a huge variety of natural foods and this is part of God's provision for us and why healthy food is so important.

However even people eating a good diet will need to take supplements because stress is a continual drain on their bodies and you can't eat enough to keep up the supply.

Stress formulas, containing multi minerals and the entire vitamin Bs, are recommended and like everything mentioned in this book can be purchased through the author's web page or clinic. Powerful herbs that calm, relax and support nervous systems are also available.

Common herbs used for stress management are;
- Zizyphus
- Passion Flower
- Magnolia
- Valerian

St. John's Wort (when necessary use separately because if you are on anti depressant it is contraindicated- don't use).

(If you are pregnant or taking any anti-depressant medication – please check with your doctor before taking any herbs.)

Herbs to help repair long term stress and sickness damage, (and boost energy by supporting adrenal function) include:
- Rehmannia
- Withania
- American Ginseng
- Astragalus

I discuss stress in more detail in my book Daniel's Diet Lifestyle.

Toxemia

Our bodies are all deteriorating and aging prematurely because of the accumulation of acids and different foreign matter within our bodies. When the liver is overloaded and its capacity to filter (detox) is lowered, many physical and even emotional problems can occur.

Toxemia (toxic overload) is one of the main reasons for degenerative disease.

Common psychological effects, in both men and women are:
- Liver/lactate induced anxiety (LIAS)
- Depression and mood swings
- Premenstrual syndrome (PMS)
- Irritability
- Tiredness
- Hormonal imbalance

This is why I believe that Daniel's Diet works on the mind and emotions, as well as the physical.

Partial fasting and supplements, like antioxidants, is a major weapon in the fight for health in mind, body and spirit.

What Are Antioxidants?

Antioxidants are a major active ingredient found in natural foods. They were designed to help neutralize and eliminate oxidants (toxins) from our bodies, and hold the balance of power between toxic overload and good health.

This is why less cancer and other types of illnesses are experienced in countries where it's customary to consume plenty of vegetables and fruit.

Natural foods contain substances that are by their nature, healing, protective and energizing. They contain life.

Every color, family and type of food has something different to offer us. The key is to eat a daily diet that contains enough quantity and variety of them.

To perceive that all natural food is life-giving, energizing, disease fighting, body balancing and flavorsome should revolutionize our lives and encourage us all to eat more of the natural food from God's Garden.

In fact, by following a healthy lifestyle and by really working at your health, every physical body has the ability to renew itself in approximately twelve months. **Every 3 months our bloodstream is renewed**

and following this all our cells are renewed. (This is why I suggest when you are taking any form of natural treatment (supplements) to take them consistently for three months minimum, and then reassess your situation). In other words – the Good News is, if you are sick or diseased at this moment and choose to change to a completely healthy lifestyle, in three months your blood and circumstances are changing, from where you are now to where you want to be (being healed). If you are sick or diseased at this moment and choose to change to a completely healthy lifestyle, your body now has the chance to self-repair and regenerate itself.

Eating fresh food grown in our local community or climate is the ideal, but modern facilities don't limit us to this. We can get fresh foods all year round. Most people eat an average of two to three vegetables a day, but it's often the same vegetables. I suggest that it would be beneficial to increase this intake and add more variety. The menu suggestions at the end of this book will enlighten you to different natural foods. Every color and variety of natural foods contains a different combination of life-giving nutrients and body balancing antioxidants.

Overeating manufactured, 'fast' (take-away) and processed foods will cause a depletion of our body's nutrient supply. We can eat regularly - even overeat - but still be undernourished. Why? Because the majority of processed foods do not contain enough of the right nutrients.

Let's face it, because of modern society and lifestyles, even those who are eating a well balanced diet would benefit from taking antioxidant supplements. Most naturopaths that I know (including myself) take them as a preventative and healing supplement.

Antioxidant Supplements:
First include a variety of natural/organic (where possible) fruit and vegetables in your diet. (You can also buy concentrated fruit and vegetables in capsules or in powder form).

- Green Tea   • Zinc

- Grape Seed Extract
- Bilberry Extract
- Vitamins C & E
- Pine Bark Extract
- Ginkgo Biloba Extract
- Resveratrol.

Although optional, one, or a combination of these, taken with vegetable juices and the liver support herbs whilst on Daniel's Diet is a lethal weapon against disease and ill health.

The Liver, Our Internal Filter System

The liver and kidneys are our internal filtration system. Our liver detoxifies and processes for excretion, all substances that circulate in our blood. This not only means pollutant chemicals absorbed from the environment, but also infective agents, food substances, drugs and the body's own waste and excess hormones. The liver processes about 2 liters of blood every minute. However, after continual overload our livers slowly but surely block up, just like any filter does. Unfortunately, we cannot change these internal filters like we can those of a car; the liver can only be cleaned by special internal cleansing. This is where Daniel's Diet comes in. It is the key to detoxing our entire body, including the liver.

I see lots of people who have allergies or sensitivities to everyday foods. These intolerances cause a daily overload of toxins, making the body a continual war zone, day in, day out, and this unrelenting fight causes tiredness and eventually a weakened immune system.

Keeping the liver healthy is vitally important and not only for those who drink alcohol. Using the Daniel's Diet three or four times a year and living a moderate and healthy lifestyle goes a long way to keeping it healthy.

Beetroot's (red beets) Role in Liver Support

Beetroot (Beets) is regarded as a blood cleanser and blood tonic. It helps our liver, gallbladder and kidneys function, by stimulating action within the liver it aids blood circulation.

Tinned beetroot is soaked in vinegar so on this diet it's not recommended. However, beetroot that is raw, steamed or juiced is recommended. Diabetics should not drink this juice because it may alter blood sugar levels.

Liver Support Supplements:

- St Mary's Thistle
- Dandelion Root
- Globe Artichoke
- Vitamin C

Most of these herbs can be purchased singularly or in different combinations containing two or more. Ideally, these herbs should be taken for two to three weeks before the start of Daniel's Diet to aid the body's adjustment to the detox. However, for those who can't wait that long to begin I suggest starting on them as soon as possible, even two or three days before will be helpful. Continue with the herbs throughout the diet and for up to three months after.

These herbs support, cleanse, stimulate, protect and regenerate the liver and assist the gall bladder. They are also helpful in overcoming high cholesterol, hormonal imbalance, digestive disorders, liver disease and, of course, help in detoxifying the body.

I recommend taking these herbs because, let's face it, we can all do with a liver cleanse. For anyone who is very toxic or has been diagnosed with health issues the above combinations will be especially beneficial. For those who have had their gall bladder removed, when used in conjunction with a natural digestive enzyme (e.g. Lipase) supplement and squeezed lemon juice, these herbs will assist your body to cope with digestion of fat and adjust to the loss of the gall bladder.

Gall Bladder:

I am amazed at the number of people coming through my clinic that have had their gall bladder removed and have never been told what that means to their future health. Sure, people live quite normally after the operation, at least to some degree. However God gave us a gall bladder for a specific reason. That is to release gall into the stomach every time we eat fatty foods to break that food down and digest it. When it's removed you lose this ability. The good news for post operation people is that there are supplements that you can ingest with meals that are fatty in nature. What this means is that you take the supplement with your meals to aid digestion, which is impeded by the removal of your gall bladder. One patient of mine said that after me telling her this information and using the supplement her whole health changed. For years after her gall bladder operation she suffered digestive and stomach problems. Bloating, excess gas, uncomfortable - painful stomach, and she couldn't sleep properly after heavy meals. Within weeks these symptoms had all gone.

Foods that will specifically aid detoxification and really goes well with this diet;
- Broccoli
- Watercress
- Pomegranate
- Turmeric
- Beetroot (Beets)
- Ginger

Detoxification support
Epsom salts baths encourage the elimination of toxins through the skin. If you can include two Epsom salt baths in the 10 days it will aid your detox. Pour 2 tablespoons of Epsom salt into your bath with lots of hot water. Epsom salts baths encourage the elimination of toxins through the skin. *Caution:* Do not take this kind of bath if you have eczema/broken skin (will sting) or high blood pressure. Dry Skin Brushing. The skin is the largest organ of the body and one of its many roles is to help excrete toxins. Skin brushing helps toxin removal by improving circulation and stimulating the lymphatic system.

Please note: I am not individually prescribing any herbs in this book, but supplying you with general information only. Daniel's Diet does not rely on taking any supplements; however as you can appreciate by now, many people need some extra assistance. If you chose not to take any supplement that's fine, just stick to the diet plan.

CHAPTER FIVE

QUICK AND HEALTHY WEIGHT LOSS

Is there such a thing as a quick and healthy weight loss diet?
YES! In my opinion, there is.

There have been many warnings about quick weight loss plans and fad diets, and rightly so. Often referred to as yo-yo diets these, if undertaken unwisely or ad hoc, can have a detrimental effect on the body. In the long term they are not only unhealthy, but can actually cause uncontrolled weight gain.

A yo-yo diet is a program that revolves around feast and famine. The result of this plan is simple - fight hunger – give up and over indulge – fight hunger.

In other words, wait as long as possible before eating or simply skip meals. Since these diets provide no set routine for eating; bingeing or overeating at the wrong times is a common event and one that is usually followed by a loss of control over food decisions.

After all, when you're starving hungry you want to eat right away, and that's when unhealthy, junk or fast food becomes an easy choice.

The danger here is the appearance of metabolism problems, the very thing you don't want – a sluggish metabolism. It also creates uncontrolled carbohydrate/sugar/fat/salt cravings. To say nothing of the more than likely weight gain, ill health, frustration, and possible depression or even bulimic tendencies. The very things the dieting was supposed to help you with in the first place.

Daniel's Diet, encourages eating five times a day. There are no set limits on the food quantities. Daniel's Diet gives a quick weight loss plan in the first ten days, and then encourages slow subsequent weight loss afterwards.

Eat as much as you like as long as you eat the right foods although, as with any diet, overeating is strongly advised against. When you are full, stop eating.

After the 10-day plan explained in this book, a lifestyle of moderation is recommended. Moderation is a key issue to maintaining weight loss and health over a long period of time. (Explained in detail in my book –'Daniel's Diet Lifestyle')

This is a diet of moderation, not laws. Nobody wants a diet that says, "You can't eat this or that for the rest of your life."

Most people want a long-term diet that is relevant to their lifestyle and one they can enjoy and relax with on a day-to-day basis. The key to finding this is first knowing the dangerous foods and choosing not to eat them very often. The second key is, understanding what moderation really means. Learn to say "NO" to your emotional or bodily desires when they try and lead you back to your old ways.

From my empirical clinical experience, I have found that on a day-to-day eating basis, most people do not have healthy, regular and balanced eating habits. The basis of this statement is indisputable as we look at the statistics for obesity and disease in our society.

In fact, I suspect that many of those who choose to follow this diet even though it's a partial fast, will find they are eating better, and more healthily, than they have been for a long time. This fact alone should alleviate any dietary and nutritional concerns people may have about doing this diet.

One question I sometimes hear from people planning to go on this weight loss program regards a concern about lack of variety and taste.

My answer to this is, first understand that Daniel's Diet is a restricted and cleansing diet. It's going to limit your normal choices – this is the whole idea! But that doesn't mean there won't be other tasty foods to eat instead.

Secondly, make the challenge of shopping fun; prepare foods you have never or rarely ever tried before. Thirdly, there are many wonderful and tasty recipes that stay within the allowed food guidelines. I have my new book out *Daniel's Diet Recipe Guide* where you will find very tasty and creative recipes to use over the 10 days.

I urge you to try this diet; only good things can come from making the changes recommended here.

Enjoy the benefits of it. Experience the extra energy, health and clarity. Feel as wonderful as the hundreds of people who have already done this diet. These people feel alive again. They are buzzing with enthusiasm because of the pounds they have dropped so quickly. They also have an increased confidence, a confidence that comes from knowing they have the power to choose their food and eating plans, rather than being controlled by them.

What If I Don't Lose Weight?

It's my experience that the majority of people who complete this diet lose weight. There are some cases, of course, where underlying factors, like a metabolism problem or organ malfunction have initially slowed the weight loss.

There are three main physical factors stopping or making it difficult for weight loss.

Insulin resistance - The modern diet is full of high glycaemic loaded foods, in other words foods loaded with sugar. When you eat high amounts of glucose or refined carbohydrates it will cause the release of high amounts of insulin, encouraging your body to store these carbohydrate foods as fat, thereby stopping fat from being used as energy, resulting in weight gain. *Losing weight becomes very difficult if you have raised insulin levels* but when your body's blood sugar and insulin levels are pushed low enough (by eating correctly) your body will respond and switch to a higher level of fat burning. This is a key to losing weight. I treat many people with both types of diabetes (1and 2) and those with

Insulin resistance and if the patient is compliant to my instructions of eating real home cooked food and cut right down on sugars and refined carbs, and increases exercise, takes specific herbs and minerals - then you see wonderful changes in their blood sugar reading. Try the herbs I mention under the heading 'Herbs for Weight Loss', later in this chapter and see the results.

I suggest you ask your Doctor for a specific 'Insulin Fasting' test as well as a glucose test, as they are different tests. If you are on medication you must work with a Doctor or Naturopath when you undertake any major changes, as you would need to monitor the diabetic medications and adjust them accordingly, as your blood sugar reading improve.

Slow Metabolism and sluggish Thyroid – see more on this next. Follow the same plan as point one with the addition of some herbs.

Hormone Imbalance – high oestrogen and low Progesterone. Often thyroid and hormone problems are found together. Use the same diet plan as the other two points and consider a saliva hormone test and or herbs to assist.

But the good news is by using the diet plans I have made and with lifestyle changes you can reverse the situation and not only lose weight but address the health issues as well.

By using the diet plans I have set for you, if you start to lose weight and see progress then all is good. If not then it simply tells you not to give up but you may have to seek professional advice. Whichever category you are in it is a win -win situation.

Anyone who follows this diet, but does not lose much or any weight should see this as a 'positive'? Why, because it is showing you that there is something else you may need to address to achieve the weight loss.

Something that is working behind the scene to harm your body and if you discover it now you can change it. Be it insulin resistance, hormone problems, low thyroid function, stress and high/low cortisol or more exercise. It should motivate you to search out and find what is holding you back, what is the cause. You may need a practitioner to help you find the answers. This will benefit you in the long term. However I can offer you much support and help you get the answers you need for losing stubborn weight.

Most times there is an explanation for what is, or isn't, happening to your body.

Most people put weight on slowly, over a period of time; too much of the wrong food and not quite enough exercise is the main reason. To achieve long-term weight loss there is one vital rule - the energy put into your body (the food) must be less than the energy used. This is a mathematical and physical law. Even a good diet may not bring a satisfactory weight loss unless the expenditure of energy is increased. This means there must be regular and consistent exercise included in your long-term lifestyle as well as the dietary changes.

Most times there is an explanation for what is, or isn't, happening to your body. And if there is ever any concern about a reaction to a certain food or supplement always use wisdom - stop taking it and seek a practitioner's advice.

Let's look at some things I can advise you on right now...

Do You Have an Under Active Thyroid Gland and a Sluggish Metabolism?

A lot of people who consult with me suspect they have a sluggish metabolism, but are not sure. The way to tell is to take notice of what your body is trying to tell you.

Signs that your thyroid is under functioning:
Weight gain – Easy weight gain, or difficulty losing weight, despite a solid exercise program and watching your diet is a strong indicator.

Reduced energy levels – Fatigue, lethargy and lack of enthusiasm is a common symptom of a low-functioning thyroid. This is also a sign of possible depression, so if you've been diagnosed with depression, you'll want to make sure your physician checks your thyroid levels.

If your thyroid is tired, you will be too. Some of the key symptoms of thyroid fatigue include:

- You lack the desire or energy to exercise, and typically not exercising on a consistent basis.
- A heavy or tired head or neck, especially in the afternoon, as your head is a very sensitive indicator of thyroid hormone status.
- Poor memory
- Falling asleep as soon as you sit down and don't have to do anything
- Sensitivity to cold – if you suffer from cold hands and feet when you normally shouldn't. Your partner may complain how cold your feet are – even in bed.
- Hair keeps falling out – I treat many women with this problem. The good news is that it is easily reversible when treated with specific herbs and nutrients.
- Dry, rough or scaly skin and dry hair.
- Constipation and unexplained indigestion.

Any of these symptoms can be indicative of an underactive thyroid, but the more of these symptoms you experience, the higher the likelihood that you have hypothyroidism.

How to test yourself for a slow metabolism & sluggish thyroid?

There is a very effective, simple home test called, Resting Basal Body Temperature Test, which measures your metabolic rate and thyroid function. If your test is low – then your weight loss will be slow (and probably your energy too). An under active thyroid gland can create a drop in body temperature. This is what the temperature test will ascertain. An over active thyroid gland can increase body temperature. Often the symptom of cold hands and feet can point towards a low thyroid function.

Before going to sleep place a thermometer next to your bed, then as soon as you wake in the morning and before you get out of bed, take your temperature by placing the thermometer under your arm for several minutes (with digital thermometers use where it stipulates; e.g. Your mouth – but not your ear as I have found this to be inaccurate). Record the temperature for four consecutive mornings and work out the average temperature over those four readings. Any starting date is appropriate for men and postmenopausal women (or for any women missing a cycle). For menstruating women the most accurate readings are taken when you start recording on the second day of menstruation. If you take your test during ovulation your body temperature will rise then because of your normal hormone elevation and not because of your thyroid. Also if you have a fever or flu don't take it then as it will give a false reading. Your Basal Body Temperature should be 36.4 degrees Celsius (97.6 Fahrenheit) or above, if it's below 36.4 degrees Celsius (97.6 Fahrenheit) it's sluggish and you'll need supplements to help restore it back to a normal level. The lower your numbers are the worse your problem is. Even small drops and readings of 36.1 or 36.2 are indicating a sluggish thyroid. I regularly see people with reading of 35.2 or there about. This is often after being for medical thyroid tests and being told that there is nothing wrong.

Remember the temperature must be taken before you get out of bed, before you eat or drink or move around in the morning. The minute you start moving around after waking up your temperature begins to rise. This test is a great help and gives a general indication of your metabolism, however it does not diagnose specific problems or override what your doctor's advice may be.

If you have had a thyroid function test from your doctor and you are told its 'normal', I suggest you still try the Resting Basal Test yourself.

Sometimes you may have a borderline low thyroid function, which may not be considered important on the doctor's test. If this is the case you may have a sluggish metabolism and not realize it. In other words your thyroid function test indicates there is nothing serious wrong with your thyroid (praise God) but it still may be under functioning or struggling to keep up with all the demands you have placed on it. This is the 'grey area' that is often overlooked and where this simple home test is invaluable.

Julia; in the following case history had a below normal resting body temperature.

Case History

Julia; (mid 30's) reported that after ten days on Daniel's Diet she had only lost 2 kg. Whilst she was feeling a lot better in herself, she was a little disappointed at not having lost as much weight as her friend had. During our consultation I discovered that Julia had an ongoing hypoglycemic problem caused by eating excess sugar and refined carbohydrate. She also had strong signs of a hormonal imbalance. Because of these I suggested Julia take her Resting Basal Body Temperature. She did so and on the second consultation she informed me it was an average of 34.8 degrees, which indicated a sluggish metabolism and thyroid gland.

Julia had completed the 10-day plan, but now needed a special diet program to suit her individuality. For her it was a high protein and low carbohydrate diet. She was not to eat any carbohydrates after lunchtime, to cut her fruit intake down to 3 pieces a day and to totally avoid fruit juices.

For the hypoglycemia I prescribed:

A formula of Chromium, Magnesium, Zinc, B12 and Folic acid, and another of Brindleberry (The fruit Garcinia Cambogia, is also called brindleberry) and Gymnema.

These wonderful minerals and herbs help stop sugar cravings, speed up metabolism and replenish the deficiencies that occur with excess sugar consumption. Hydroxycitric acid in Brindleberry helps in achieving weight loss.

For the hormone imbalance I prescribed:
• Vitex Agnus-Castus (also called Chaste Tree), Dong Quai and B6 to assist the hormonal balance.

For her sluggish metabolism and thyroid gland I prescribed:
*   Potassium iodide, zinc, combined with specific herbs and minerals to support thyroid and adrenal function. (She also undertook a Hair Mineral Analysis, which helped me be more specific on prescribing for her).
*   Kelp & Tyrosine (an amino acid) to stimulate her thyroid function.

(If you are taking thyroid medication avoid taking kelp and Tyrosine, as this may interfere with the medication, ask your doctor).

Liver Support Herbs - to help eliminate excess hormones accumulating in the blood:

This herbal combination was given to support the detoxifying capacity of the liver and increase bile flow to maintain natural body waste elimination: Milk Thistle, Globe artichoke, Curcumin and Broccoli sprout powder.

During the 10-day diet Julia was also taking a special mixed herb called 'Fibre Blend' (AIM), which includes Psyllium husks. This mixture, she kept taking because fibre was very important in the overall scheme, it helped to mop up (absorb and eliminate) excess sugars and to keep her bowels regular. This supplement aids the whole health and detoxification process. Psyllium husks on its own is a great fibre and relatively cheap. After these changes Julia started losing weight. Taking the holistic approach of treating the whole body with diet, exercise and supplements enabled us to discover and treat her individual needs.

To the uninitiated taking this amount of supplements may seem a little excessive.

If initially one specific supplement is required for each problem area, then regrettably there will be many. In the above case, if only one area had been treated Julia would probably not have received the results she was hoping for. It is vital to treat all the areas of the body that have been damaged through previous lifestyle and food choices.

I have many other case histories where stubborn weight loss was overcome by diet alone. If you are not sure if you need to take supplements, I suggest you do the diet without any and see what happens. If you are content with the results and can follow a healthy lifestyle in the long term, great! If you see there is more to be achieved, then do the diet again and use the herbs this time.

What? No Weighing Foods or Counting Calories?

I have never weighed or measured foods. I find it too much trouble, so I rarely ask others to do it. People who are familiar with measuring food might find it helpful in the early stages of this diet but, in the long term, it shouldn't be necessary. If you enjoy following charts and counting calories then, of course, stick to what helps you as an individual.

Personally, I have found that setting too many rules and regulations can cause people to spend too much time thinking about food. In my opinion, this is often why diets that list what can and cannot be eaten tend not to work over long periods of time, they become too hard to maintain. Planning wisely, sharing knowledge and enjoying a healthy lifestyle is a great thing to do, and a 'healthy' topic of conversation but putting too much emphasis on food may lead to fanaticism, bingeing, bulimia and yo-yo dieting.

For a diet to have longevity and to be successful, the lifestyle needs to be enjoyable and easy to adhere to. A Moderation Diet, which I recommend after the completion of Daniel's Diet 10-day plan, offers this (see my book Daniels Diet Lifestyle). In simple terms it's a diet founded on the theories of Daniel's Diet but it includes a variety of more everyday foods - including healthy meats and the occasional treat and feast. For example, when eating meat, the size of a good portion is measured by the size of the palm of your hand.

By the end of this book people who are used to being told (or are telling themselves) how many kilojoules, fats or calories to eat, will hopefully have learned why to eat or not eat certain foods and know that a general idea of quantity is good enough, because now they are eating with wisdom and choosing to eat foods that are good.

Daniel's Way Diet - a Partial Fast

Daniel's Diet is different from most other diets in that it's a partial fast for a set amount of time. A fast requires eating no food. A partial fast on the other hand allows unlimited (with wisdom) amounts of specified or selective food.

This principle of partial fasting can become a good short-term discipline and thereby a great help in the long-term goal of longevity of diet and weight control. Especially after harmful foods have been recognized and rejected. Fasting is an overlooked and underestimated principle in today's society.

The purpose of the partial fast is multiple:
- to lose weight and detoxify the body
- to recognize harmful foods
- to feel good
- to get control of overeating
- to give up cigarettes and harmful substances
- to change a health situation
- to seek spiritual help or direction in any area you choose

The everyday changes may mean having to learn to cook and present meals a different way, but once the effort and alterations are made they will integrate into part of a daily routine. The cost of eating this way should average out to about the same as before. You will be spending more in some areas but less in others. During the actual Daniel's Diet you should save money as you are not buying many foods for the 10 days.

Every routine you followed pre-diet was new at some time, it had to be taught, learnt and followed - this is no different.

Regaining Control

There may well be an inner struggle in anyone who wants to complete this diet. Some people will start into the 10 days and, for various reasons, stop before the designated time.

If this should be you, my advice is don't feel guilty; there are plenty more opportunities in your future to come back and have another go. Always keep your resolve to achieve health and happiness, don't let anything interfere with that. Any change from your present way of eating is going to be beneficial to you. Giving up or cutting right down on any harmful food like soda or chocolate for example will help your health in the short term and long term.

The beauty of this diet plan is that you can come back to it at any time and even three, five or six days on this program achieves good results. So, relax. Prepare yourself over whatever length of time you need and when you are ready, start the diet again. The results will be worthy of your effort and determination to finish.

I have had people attend my weekly teachings for months before they eventually gather up the willpower to do the diet. Others start straight away, do it for two or three days and repeat this every few weeks until they are ready to finish the entire ten days.

Daniel set two precedents for what I would call partial fasting - one in Daniel, Chapter 1 and the other in Chapter 10: 2-3. Fasting is a very powerful process or principle and is becoming a lost art within the church and society. An indication of the importance of fasting is that it is mentioned in the Bible over seventy times.

Jesus Himself expects us to fast. He said, *"When I am gone (resurrected) then they shall fast, in these days."* (Luke 5:35) This tells us that fasting is good for us, and we should be doing it more often. Daniel's diet offers you the perfect partial fasting technique. It can help you break the 'Emotional Eating' hold that influences your life.

A whole new world awaits – enjoy.

Gooey Fat Cells

Excess weight is not just a bit of inert fat, sitting around our middle but a biological active tissue that is toxic. In fact, fat is a remarkably active substance. 'Love handles' are not cute they are toxic waste dumps. Excess fat cells behave like our endocrine cells, constantly producing and secreting a wide variety of hormones and other so called growth factors into the bloodstream. These substances send signals to other parts of the body, and it is these signals that, under certain conditions, seem to make it easier for toxic by-products to initiate, and to grow.

An example of this is that obese women who have had a hysterectomy or are in menopause can and do still produce estrogen, from their fat cells. Obese women in general are often estrogen dominant (some men too, especially if they have a fat gut and have grown 'man boobs') because their fat cells and poor diet are creating too much estrogen. This creates hormonal imbalance.

Try to visualize your gooey fat cells.

They are like small, sticky bubbles clumping together, mostly around your thighs, heart and stomach. If you are overweight, sticky masses of these fat cells begin to join together and misshape your body. Imagine how every time you eat excess animal fat, sugar, chocolate, refined carbohydrates, deep-fried or junk foods these fat cells multiply. However, by changing to Daniel's Diet, the multiplication of gooey fat cells not only stops but the cells slowly begin to break off and reduce in number; resulting in a slimmer you. Picture in your mind your body as it is now.

See yourself eating healthy foods and enjoying them. See the fat cells breaking off. Picture in your mind the body you want to have. Know that you are becoming slimmer and healthier because of your choices and because of the good food you are eating and the exercise you are undertaking.

Drink plenty of water. When enough water travels through the blood, it reaches the fat cells, lubricates the area and starts to help the cells un-glue, flushing them back into the body's elimination system. By exercising at the same time the body is able to burn up the released fat as energy. These two lifestyle habits, together with regular bowel movements, enable the body to eliminate all the excess fat and waste. This is the way to win the war against the bulge and toxic overload.

Back to the image of your ideal body.

You have just drunk your glass of water; you have been for a forty-minute walk in the park or along a beach to get your exercise and balance your negative to positive ion ratio. So not only have those struggling fat cells now broken free but they've also been burnt up as energy. You go to the scales and the dial doesn't go round quite so far. You look at yourself in the mirror and smile. Hallelujah - The plan is working. You go to the wardrobe and get out your favorite pair of jeans. The ones you've not been able to zip up. You grin as the zipper now glides up with ease. Pretty soon, you think, you'll be giving them away to someone else who needs this book! Your real self and your visual picture are beginning to merge.

Visualization becomes action. Action becomes a reality.

7 Secrets to Losing Weight

Daniel's Way to Weight Loss will give you the foundation and starting point to kick start a new healthy lifestyle. **These Seven secrets will give you the keys to long term health and weight management.**

What is the missing link for you? Like my old herbalist mentor used to say, "What I tell you now is worth more than gold."

To beat any fat cells that may be bunching together to form excess fat and cellulite it's vital that the following seven points are adopted into your regular lifestyle. Understanding this first point especially will change your life!

1. Eat a diet low in sugar and refined carbohydrate and increase good quality protein.

Nature has provided us three main sources of energy. Our body can burn stored fat, glucose (carbohydrate), or protein. If you eat less carbohydrate than you require for energy, then your stored fat is burned to provide your body's energy requirements. This means you should lose weight if you use the right order of eating, and the idea is to restrict the one which your body chooses as its first source; which is sugars or carbohydrates and your body then has to burn the second one (fat) for energy. Of course fat is the one you want dissolved to lose weight and this is the plan to do just that.

As this point is so important let me repeat it another way to make it clear. Your body will use carbohydrates as its first option of burning up energy/fuel. So it stands to reason that if you cut right back on refined carbohydrates in your diet and eat less than you require for energy, then your body's stored fat is burned to provide you with your necessary energy requirements.

This means you should lose weight, but most importantly, in the long term you will not put any more weight back on. This comes about because you are restricting the first fuel system your body will use, which is sugars and carbohydrates, and this forces your body to burn your stored fat for fuel.

Continual Hunger: Eating too many refined carbohydrates will cause you to have a big appetite and to have sweet cravings. Even after finishing a meal, you know you can't be hungry so soon and yet your body is still not satisfied. You keep looking for the sweets. If this is you, then all you need to do to overcome these cravings is to eat less sugar and refined cab.

Keep in mind that most people eat too much refined carbohydrates in their daily diet and this will lead to obesity over years. This is why a lot of people 'yo-yo' diet. The minute they finish a (any) diet plan they go back to eating too much refined carbohydrates, so they put all the weight back on and the cycle continues.

The modern diet is full of sugar. The following foods are refined carbs – food such as starchy, highly processed bread, packet cereal, white flour products, cakes, cookies (biscuits), ice cream, pastry, pasta, white rice, fast foods, don't forget alcohol and sugary products such as soft drinks, cordials and reconstituted fruit juices are all quickly converted by your body into sugar (glucose). High amounts of glucose will cause the release of high amounts of insulin, encouraging your body to store carbohydrates as fat and stop fat being used as energy (therefore increasing weight gain).

Although vegetables and fruit contain carbohydrates they are classed as 'complex' and not included in the dangerous sugar variety which are 'simple' or 'refined' carbohydrates.

This 10 day health plan will help many lose weight quickly. It will help detox your body and get you motivated to continue long term weight loss and a healthy lifestyle. My goal is to offer you strategies that will help you lose weight and gain good health.

On this specific diet plan, protein is NOT from animals but found in legumes and pulses, brown rice, sea vegetables, miso, tofu, tempeh, almonds, pistachios, walnuts, brazil nuts, split peas, chickpeas, lentils, seeds and the bean family. After the 10 days on this diet and if you are undertaking my 'The 6 week Low Carb Diet' – you will be adding fish (with scales), lean meats, chicken, turkey, eggs, tofu, goat cheese/ milk etc.

2. Drink two quarts (2 liters, 9 cups) of water a day.
The average body loses about 2 quarts of water each day through normal elimination and perspiration/evaporation. This must be replenished daily. This means water only, not counting your veggie juices. Green tea is counted in the 2 liters.

3. Maintain regular bowel movements.
This should be approximately two eliminations per day. If not then consider using an herbal laxative or Epson salts for the ten days, not long term as your bowel needs to work regularly on its own natural action (peristalsis). I talk more on this later on this chapter under constipation.

4. Don't eat late at night and eat slowly.
An evening meal should be light on the stomach and containing no carbohydrates. Avoid late evening snacks. If you do have to eat late make sure it's non-fattening foods and definitely not a carbohydrate or sugar. Eat slowly and not in front of the T.V. By wolfing down our food we increase the risk of gaining weight. By eating too fast and until feeling full overrides the signals in the brain that normally encourage self-control and consequently not eating as much. By watching TV we are not concentrating on the amount of food we consume and we can just go on nibbling away even when not hungry.

5. Don't overeat.
The original reason for weight gain is still valid. If more food is eaten than energy burned off, you have to gain weight – it's a physical and mathematical law. Especially at night, you don't want to be eating a large meal in the evening and then sit and do no exercise, go to bed and still no exercise to burn off the food you ate for dinner. Common sense tells you that weight must be gained if you do this, as well as having a poor quality of sleep.

6. The Importance of Exercise – There are no short cuts. No one can do it for you, and it must be done, so decide to get in the habit regularly and enjoy. If you exercise before a meal this will give your body the opportunity to burn the stored fat as well and help you lose weight. There is no doubt it is a vital ingredient to weight loss, health, vitality and energy.

Exercise has many health benefits including aiding digestion and elimination.

It helps us cope with stress. It puts oxygen back into our blood. And, by pushing toxins out through our perspiration, it clears what would otherwise sit under the surface of our skin causing toxic overloads in our body, especially on the Lymphatic system. Sweat is very beneficial in helping our bodies eliminate poisons and toxins.

During the 10 days of this health plan you only need to exercise gently. A minimum of 30 minutes exercise each day is your goal. Walking, swimming or whatever exercises you enjoy are all excellent ways to support your detoxification process. If you are fit and healthy and used to eating a restricted diet, then exercise as much as you feel like.

For others who may be obese, have a poor diet leading to commencing this program or have very high levels of stress (adrenal fatigue) try to avoid strenuous exercise whilst on the 10 days, as your body needs to keep its energy focused on cleansing and healing.

Some overweight people find it hard to exercise. I know lots of people feel that they just don't have the energy to do it. This, sadly, causes a 'Catch 22' situation. After all, if you don't exercise, you won't burn up fat stores and regain energy. Yet, if you don't regain your energy how will exercising become any easier or any more fun? This feeling of apathy has to be overcome. There can be no excuses. Start slowly then build up a progressive momentum. Even five minutes a day will help at the start. Then, as fitness improves, build up to forty-five minutes or more. Initially you may have to force yourself to start exercising but afterwards you'll always feel better. Exercise releases 'feel good' hormones called endorphins, once you become regular at it. (Anyone with severe injuries, heart problems, high blood pressure or body pain should follow the instructions of their physiotherapist or doctor.)

After exercising it's wise to eat something nutritious within half an hour completion as you need to replace lost energy and prevent the overwhelming cravings of sugar or carbs' that often drives us to heading for chocolate or any convenient junk food or sweet fix that manifests itself.

Increasing weight bearing exercise as well as aerobic is the best plan. This gives you more muscle mass and will increase your metabolism. A higher metabolic rate helps lessen the chance for weight gain and obesity throughout life. Also, fun and active outings decrease boredom and time available for extra snacking or grazing at home. It will also help boost self-esteem and if you are an emotional eater this is a big help. Your goals need to be; realistic, enjoyable, specific, and positive.

I have found a basic heart rate monitor to be very helpful because it showed me that I was not exercising adequately. It gave me new goals to reach. In fact my heart rate was way too low to effectively burn up enough energy to lose much weight. You see its best to keep your heart rate up to a certain level (if needed get professional help to know where your individual rate should be) and for 30 – 45 minutes at a time. Then you will see better results. Also I learnt that it's more effective to vary the intensity of the aerobic exercise from moderate to high, during the work out.

Personally, I walk for an hour every second day, as well as doing stretches, sit-ups and I warm down on a mini trampoline. On alternate days I ride my push bike (a gift from a satisfied client) for 45 plus minutes.

Exercise should raise your pulse rate no more than 220 minus your age

For example:
220 – 44 years of age
176 per minute

Adequate range is 120-140 beats per minute.

Lastly, don't procrastinate. Do it now. Exercising is not an option – it's a must.

Learn to say "no" to temptation and "stop" when feeling full.

Remember, eat slowly and at the table and not in front of TV is wise. Try not to have danger foods like sweets and refined carbs' in the house. Remove the temptation.

Note: Emotional eating and stress are strong drivers of poor eating choices and consequent weight gain and are so important in the battle of losing weight. I have personally battled with this myself, so understand the very real and strong force these factors are. I know one diet does not fit all in weight loss, however this Biblical based diet is the diet plan everyone should undertake for their health.

Constipation

I never cease to be amazed at the lack of knowledge people have regarding their bowel movements. The majority of my patients do not know, and many have not even thought about, what a normal bowel motion is. I become extremely concerned when a patient tells me that they evacuate once a week or once every two to three days. Even if their doctor or Aunt Florence informs them that this is normal for their constitution, it's an absolute fallacy and dangerous to anyone who believes it.

Ideally, we should all have one to three bowel movements a day. Just like healthy babies, we should pass a motion after each meal. This natural occurrence of 'one meal in and one meal out' will leave no time for toxic overload and no build up of excess pressure or stretching and sagging of the abdomen. This normal transit time of waste through the bowel means less toxins and less disease. It's as simple as that. Being aware of this is the first step towards normal bowel activity.

Common complaints caused by constipation are, in varying degrees:
- Tiredness
- Recurring illness
- Skin problems
- Hemorrhoids (piles)
- Toxic overload
- Headaches
- Bloating
- Irritability
- Weight gain
- Poor concentration
- Diverticulosis (pouches or ballooning of the colon)

I advise people to go to the toilet whenever they feel the urge. Even if the urge isn't strong, I suggest they sit on the toilet anyway, letting their mind get used to the idea. It's very important that we give ourselves time to evacuate. Thinking about the need and being aware of its importance will help elimination become easier and more regular. Some people may need to squat on the toilet or massage their abdomen to help the process. It may even be necessary for some adults to get up ten minutes earlier in the morning to give themselves enough time to relax before they 'go'.

High fiber diets are very necessary, so is exercise and drinking plenty of clean water. Fruit and vegetables are the best form of fiber, especially for those who are sensitive to grains. To increase fiber content, eat fresh fruit and vegetables, with the skins left on. Any green leafy vegetables, like spinach or kale, are a daily necessity.

Most animal products do not contain fluid or fiber. Only foods from God's garden do. Watermelon, for example, contains clean water and lots of nutrients. It's a natural diuretic, so incorporating this fruit in your diet is recommended. Melons are best eaten on their own. This way the body can assimilate all their benefits without other foods interfering in the digestive process.

I find that most people tend to hold back going to the toilet when they're out, at school or work for example. This social way of thinking is just as detrimental to the bowel as overeating can be. It's often the pre-programming of our mind that stops people from feeling comfortable about using work, school or public toilets. The thought of hygiene is a common reason for feeling uncomfortable; a solution to this is putting down a double row of toilet paper on the seat. These are concerns that have to be resolved for your health. Remember going to the toilet is a natural habit. Everyone has to do it. Mothers should encourage dirty diapers. Teachers should make it easy for students to get out of class for toilet breaks, just as employers make it easy for employees.

Going to the bathroom should never be put off because we are stressed, preoccupied, people conscious or too busy. You see, our minds are so strong that it can mentally control our natural bowel function to fit in around our lives. Thank God, we haven't got the same control over our heartbeat and breathing. What a huge mess we'd all be in then!

It can be said that constipation is a disease of civilization but, if we understand the bowels operation and importance, it is easy to 'eliminate' the problem.

The Main Culprits

White bread, refined flour products, fatty meat, junk food/take ways, fried food, cheese/all dairy and pork are all suspect foods when it comes to constipation.

Case History

A young mother brought her nine year old daughter to see me because she wouldn't go to the toilet more than once every four or five days. The girl was so busy playing, watching TV, etc. that she just wouldn't sit on the toilet long enough for anything to happen. Natural laxatives were recommended to ease the immediate problem but they were obviously not the long-term solution. Books and comics were placed by the toilet in an effort to keep the daughter on the toilet but with only minor success. The next idea was to place the TV in front of the doorway. It worked. She learnt to sit still long enough to have regular bowel movements. It took a little time and ingenuity but it worked.

Obviously it wasn't the ideal solution, but it did work. (The TV was taken away after a short period of time).

Alleviating Constipation

Recipe: Soak five or more prunes overnight in pure squeezed lemon juice.

Next morning, drink the juice and eat the prunes.

This recipe is a wonderful way to start the day and gives an idea on how we can help ourselves. But, everyone responds differently to stimuli, so find the one that suits you best.

Taking the liver cleansing supplement will especially help those with a long term clogged system and obesity.

Laxatives

Natural Laxatives are good for short-term use only and eating natural foods containing fiber is the more ideal way to ensure we 'go' naturally, once or twice a day.

For those who need a laxative during this diet, large doses of Magnesium are my first recommendation. Select a magnesium oxide powder and take a teaspoonful in water twice daily until the bowels loosen - (ask at the store where you purchase it, for any details if you are unsure of which supplement is best). Include one heaped teaspoon of Vitamin C powder taken with or soon after the magnesium. It is also very good as a laxative and works the same way as the magnesium. They both compliment the detox program very well.

Once the bowels have been activated, stop or slow down the dose to once daily then build it up again the next day if needed to get the same results. Stop when the fiber included in the rest of the diet starts to work, you become regular and everything works naturally. Don't use if abdominal pain, nausea or vomiting is present.

For extra dietary roughage I would recommend Psyllium Husks since it is wheat free. Rice bran is gluten free, less harsh on your bowel and is a good alternative. One or both of these is recommended on Daniel's Diet.

Psyllium Husks are available at most health stores. Psyllium Husks will form a mucilaginous substance, which is excellent for picking up any waste material that's clinging to the bowel wall. It acts like an internal broom on the impacted waste. However, if you have been constipated for a long time don't take psyllium until your bowel is moving regularly as it does swell up when you ingest it and you don't want to block up even more. Also you must drink a large glass of water after taking it to ensure its proper action. At my clinic I use a special combination of Psyllium and several herbs, mixed to do a thorough cleaning and healing action on the intestines and bowel.

Aloe Vera Juice can also be helpful in regulating the bowels.

In stubborn cases 0.7 −1.0 fluid ounce (20-30 ml) of medicinal castor oil on an empty stomach is a good old-fashioned purgative, but because of the body's strong reaction, it's wise not to venture too far away from the toilet. During the ten days of this diet it should only be necessary to use the castor oil method one or two times.

If you have really stubborn bowels seek help from a naturopath or doctor.

Case History

Karen D (not Karen M who was in hospital) –but mentioned earlier as the lady who encouraged me to research the link between food and ME; (aged 37) was a housewife, full time secretary and helped her husband with his business. She was medically diagnosed with ME (Myalgic Encephalomyelitis/ Chronic Fatigue Syndrome).

Her symptoms included:

- *Losing interest in life*
- *Depression*
- *Extreme lethargy*
- *Severe headaches*
- *Bloating*

- *'Foggy' head*
- *Tired all the time*
- *Severe PMS*
- *Loss of sex drive*

It was evident, after only a short time of talking to Karen, that counseling for stress and dietary habits should be my first priority.

I was amazed to note that during the consultation, Karen said she evacuated her bowel 'once per week' - every Friday night when work had finished and she could relax. Immediately this struck me as a major key factor in her predicament. Previous doctors had not asked about her bowel movements choosing instead to give her antibiotics and painkillers, which had only aggravated the problem.

Karen had unconsciously developed the constipation problem herself through social tension. Whilst spending long hours at work, Karen had chosen to ignore her body's request, refusing to go to the toilet. At night she was too busy with her children and husband, then later she was just too tired to 'go.' I started Karen on Daniel's Diet, with juices and supplements.

In the initial stages she took:

1. A probiotic formula containing Lactobacillus Acidophilus and Bifidobacteria to replenish her bowels/intestines with essential bacteria.
2. Herbs for liver and bile support: St Mary's Thistle, Globe Artichoke and Bupleurum
3. Vitamin C and Magnesium (powder) in large doses to activate

the bowel and start her cleansing/detox.

Due to the severity of her circumstances, I kept Karen on the diet for three weeks, with weekly check-ups. At the end of the first week, her headaches were not as severe or often and her bowels were gradually beginning to unblock.

In the third week a herbal supplement designed for bowel cleansing, containing Psyllium husks mixed with other herbs (called Herbal Fiber Blend (AIM), available from my web site) was added to her program. I hadn't added this at the start of the diet because the Psyllium fiber would only have made the problem worse. It's important with constipation to activate the bowel before you include supplement fiber. However, once her bowels were loosened the fiber supplement replaced the high doses of vitamin C and Magnesium. By now, the continual headaches had gone and her bowels were greatly improved. She was now evacuating every second day.

By the fourth week, her bowels moved every day. Karen was feeling so good that she could hardly believe it. She has regained her energy and her concentration was back to normal levels. She was then able to slowly include fish and more whole grains into her diet and generally use the Moderation Diet principles recommended for after Daniel's Diet.

It is also worth noting Karen had made the wise decision of cutting down on her work load and she let go of trying to be "super women" and gave herself permission to have some time for herself. She learnt to say NO at the appropriate times. This way she could set her new lifestyle boundaries in place. One being that she arranged to cut her six days a week down to four and a half, which was very beneficial to her recovery.

Between the fifth and eighth week on the diet and lifestyle plan Karen said, "I feel as good now as I did when I was a teenager!"

All her energy and enthusiasm for life had returned. Where as previously she had been neglecting her husband, family and home, she was now enjoying them. She had no more PMS and her sex drive had returned. Karen's stress level had eased considerably. Her ear pain was gone (something she had forgotten to mention initially). She also said the change of diet had probably saved her marriage. And now I 'have a friend for life.'

The Emotional Link

During my years of counseling I have noticed people who refuse to let go of the past often have an emotional link to constipation. Often some form of fear, a continual anxiety in their minds, usually created by past or present circumstances. They can be holding onto old relationships or situations that give them pain or regret. People who have one or more unfinished situations in their life are often constipated and improve automatically when that situation is concluded. Improvement will come in these situations with a 'letting go' of the past and also organizing them to finish a task, to achieve something they have been wanting for a time, find accomplishment in job or personal areas and success in immediate goals.

For anyone who feels that this might relate to them I suggest making decisions and acting on them. I also suggest you learn to relax more and enjoy the journey. Also meditate on the Scriptures, Philippians 3:12-14 & 4:6-7.

Understanding True Hunger

Have you ever thought you were so starving hungry that you could 'eat a horse', but gone on to satisfy your hunger by eating just a small sandwich?

In that situation you hadn't really needed any more than that small amount. Yet, if you hadn't eaten the healthy sandwich you could have gone to a fast food restaurant and ordered two hamburgers, large fries and a large soda instead. What's more, you would have eaten the lot and no doubt had an ice cream to follow. Why is that?

It's because we often don't eat just to satisfy our natural physiological hunger. And the above kinds of foods, due to their soft texture, fat, salt/sugar content and half-warm temperature tend to make us eat too fast and too much.

Recognizing true hunger sensations and not confusing them with abnormal cravings is essential. Stomach hunger is a natural, empty, hollow sensation and the buildup of stomach acid will create a growl or rumbling sensation. This signals that the body requires food.

Eating before this sensation occurs, keeps overloading our body with excess food and does not allow the body to burn its stored fuel (fat deposits). Any new fuel (food) put into the body will be utilized first, especially carbohydrates, leaving the fat cells sitting there not used and growing bigger with every mouthful of excess food. When it's time to refuel, eat something, but eat only enough to satisfy the hunger.

Eating slowly is the key; because our appetite for food is satisfied by a mechanism triggered inside our brain sending a "stop eating, I'm full" message via the stomach.

From when we start eating it takes twenty minutes or more for the brain to receive the not hungry signal from our stomach. **This means, if we eat our meal in ten minutes it will be ten more minutes before we feel satisfied. Which is plenty of time for us to consume enormous quantities of unnecessary food? Slow down!**

Accept that it's okay to leave some food on your plate. It amazes me the amount of people who have a problem with this. It obviously comes from childhood teaching and if it's causing you to overeat – let it go. It's not going to help any of those starving children. However, the money saved on the weekly grocery bill will. It's okay to tell yourself, your parents, your grandparents, or your friends that you're full and not going to eat unnecessarily.

This is a key to Daniel's Diet, initially changing a regular pattern and an old way of thinking. Some people may currently have a routine that involves eating on the run, eating out, picking up fast food, buying prepacked or processed foods. Try changing these to habits of sitting down to enjoy home style meals. This will allow the body to absorb all the nutrients before burning them off. Never eat when angry or in a hurry – because then the body won't digest the food properly.

Herbs for Weight Loss

First I suggest you add this list of herbs to your Daniels Way diet as they all have weight losing power and quite easily be added to your cooking.

- Turmeric
- Mustard
- Ginger
- Black pepper
- Cinnamon
- Cayenne pepper
- Cardamom (aromatic spice)
- Green Tea - with a squeeze of lemon. Green tea helps your abdominal fat loss [1] [2]. It's a very good addition to this diet and general lifestyle. Drink 3 cups per day (preferably organic green tea). Herbal supplements containing Green Tea extract are often used for weight loss, but I would not recommend this as it is a concentrated source of caffeine and may be too much of a stimulant, for some people. Just to be clear; drinking 3-4 cups of green tea daily has many health benefits and it does contain caffeine but the small amounts in organic green tea is beneficial to your health and will give you a natural energy boost (you should not compare it to processed coffee). In also aids heart health by improving both blood flow and the ability of your arteries to relax.

Second consider herbal supplements that can help weight loss and stop food cravings?

Do not be misled by over the top advertising which says all you have to do is take an herbal supplement and your weight will just 'melt away'; that is fantasy and looking for the easy way out. You still have to eat less junk food and exercise.

However, concentrated good quality herbs can assist in weight loss. They encourage miracles but are not miracle workers. It's too much to expect that by merely adding an herb to a diet, weight will simply fall off. If only!

On the other hand for those serious about weight loss, those who are going to do Daniel's Diet and change old habits then, yes, the herbs will be of great benefit.

But to get the best out of any supplement it is important to:
- Know which ones to take for each individual situation.
- Know what they are for and what they do.
- Commit to taking them constantly for at least three months.
- Take the correct daily dose and read the label for any warnings.

Sometimes people ask me why their supplements aren't working and when I find out that they have only been taking one capsule a day even though the recommended dosage is three to four, the answer is obvious.

Another reason can be because they are taking an off the counter supplement that, for modern day convenience and marketing strategy recommends one tablet a day when in reality the dose needed to get the full benefit is one tablet two or three times daily. It can depend on the quality of the brand or the dosage amount in each capsule. Some cheaper brands may have very small amount of the herb in each capsule and that is why it is cheap.

Some people may suffer from poor digestion and this interferes with the absorption of the supplement, in which case a liquid form should be taken to get the best results.

Also remember the reaction is not immediate, so be prepared to take the supplements for months at a time. I usually tell my patients to aim for three months and in that time you should notice the difference.

There are herbs for every occasion! I often state in my lectures that herbs are Gods medicine and a gift to us to use when and where necessary. If you are new to the use of herbs as medicine, welcome to the ever-growing amount of enlightened people worldwide who use this method of treatment. Herbs are Gods natural medicine especially designed for our benefit.

How the Herbs Help

Some herbs reduce energy intake by decreasing appetite and reducing cravings. Other herbs increase energy expenditure by mobilizing fats or increasing metabolism. If you combine these herbs with others that boost stamina, to facilitate exercise, you have an effective herbal regime for weight loss. These combinations are especially helpful for anyone who finds it hard to lose weight, has deficiencies, cravings or other physical problems.

When these herbs are combined with exercise and lifestyle changes, expect to get results. And let's face it; any help is appreciated in the battle for health and weight loss.

As stated earlier, each individual is uniquely different and needs specific herbs for their circumstance. In this book I am not prescribing supplements for any individual but merely explaining which are appropriate and helpful in different situations. I see herbs as part of God's provision for us, so why not use them?

BRINDLEBERRY also known as Garcinia Cambogia and Malabar Tamarind

The Malabar Tamarind is commonly used in India and South-east Asia as a condiment, especially in curries. The Brindleberry fruit, which contains high levels of beneficial Hydroxycitric acid (HCA), exhibits a distinctively sweet acid taste and a unique purple color. It's sometimes used in India to make the food more 'filling and satisfying'.

Brindle Berry works as an appetite suppressant and metabolic stimulant by converting excess carbohydrate stored in the body and moving it out of the body. This herb works very well with the mineral Chromium.

CAPSICUM (Cayenne)

The cayenne or chili pepper (capsicum) is receiving much attention from scientists because of several useful medicinal properties. Cayenne significantly boosts BMR (Basal Metabolic Rate).

Research at the University of Tasmania found that a small amount of chili sauce increased the BMR in four out of six male volunteers. When fifteen people who had been on a calorie-controlled diet added chili sauce, cayenne pepper, mustard and other spices to their diet, weight loss increased by 25 per cent.

Fast Fact: by adding red and black pepper, ginger and chillies to your food you can help speed up your metabolism

FOENICULUM VULGARE (Fennel)

Fennel is regarded as an appetite suppressant in traditional medicine. The next time you are feeling hungry, try chewing a small handful of fennel seeds or drinking a cup of fennel tea and see the effect. William Cole in 'Nature's Paradise' (1650), wrote: 'Fennel is much used in drinks and broths for those that are grown fat, to abate their unwieldiness and cause them to grow more gaunt and lank.'

The ancient Greeks called fennel, Marathon, which means, 'to grow thin.' Fennel seeds are free of sugar but taste sweet due to their content of Anethole. Whether this sweet taste plays a role in their ability to suppress appetite is not known, but Anethole does chemically resemble adrenalins that stimulate metabolism and suppress appetite.

FUCUS VESICULOSIS – Bladderwrack (is a form or kelp and often sold as 'Kelp' in the health stores and pharmacies).

Bladderwrack (Fucus) is common brown seaweed rich in iodine, which is known to stimulate the thyroid gland. Stimulation of the thyroid gland increases the Basal Metabolic Rate (BMR). The BMR is the speed at which your body burns energy whilst resting. This is why bladderwrack has a wonderful reputation to help weight loss.

Contraindication: anyone taking Thyroxin or thyroid medications should avoid taking Kelp/Bladderwrack as the medications and herbs may interact negatively.

GYMNEMA – The sugar destroyer

If you have a 'sweet tooth,' this is the herb for you, along with the trace mineral Chromium. I use this herb regularly in my clinic to help overcome sugar cravings and balance blood sugar levels.

COLEUS - Coleus forskohlii:

It not only helps 'burn up' your gooey fat cells but assists your thyroid and metabolism.

Coleus extract is commonly recommended for treating hypothyroidism, a condition in which the thyroid gland produces too little thyroid hormone. Forskolin is believed to stimulate the release of thyroid hormone, thus relieving such hypothyroidism symptoms as fatigue, depression, weight gain, and dry skin

An extract of the plant Coleus has been used for centuries in herbal medicine to treat various diseases such as hypothyroidism and heart disease.

NB. I am not prescribing these herbs; I am opening your thoughts up to the possibilities that are available. Everyone is different and therefore you need individual diagnosis. However if you need help with any of these herbal protocols please contact me.

CHAPTER SIX

ARE YOU AN EMOTIONAL EATER?

How do you react to emotional problems?

If you feel lost, hurt or misunderstood, do you turn to food? Especially the kind of food you know is wrong or bad for you.

This is called comfort eating. It means using food to cover up the pain of an underlying issue that really needs to be addressed. Comfort eating is a form of codependency or escapism and a form of tranquillizer self-medication.

Unless the underlying issue that triggers an emotional eating reaction is addressed, food will constantly have a strong hold on your life.

There are numerous different issues that can cause this situation, but they can usually be put under one of three headings, or sometimes a combination of the three.

They are: physical, emotional or spiritual hurt or lack.

Problems with weight and illness are not always just about eating the wrong foods. Eating habits can be intricately intertwined with our emotions and even our spiritual well-being.

An over dependency on food or anything obsessive can be a barrier between each of us reaching an abundant, fulfilling life.

It's time to break the cycle.

Using Food as a Tranquillizer

In trying to find a way to bring the pain of some of life's experiences down to a bearable level, many people turn to a narcotic agent that will anaesthetize their pain. Everybody reacts differently, some turn to alcohol or drugs, for others it's sex or even shopping. And for many, whether they know it or not, it's food. Whenever there is a trigger for fear, anxiety, stress, anger, frustration, boredom or emotional lack or pain, they eat.

Food can be a tranquillizer and don't fool yourself, it can be every bit as addictive and detrimental as the other options. The main difference here though is that food is a socially, morally and legally acceptable way of handling stress and pain. Even Church groups label eating food as the 'acceptable sin,' with sweets and junk food available at nearly all their functions.

How Does Food Tranquillize?

Blood sugar levels rise upon the consumption of junk or sugary food. Eating them stimulates different neurochemicals (endorphins) in the brain, which have the effect of natural painkillers, relaxants and pleasure stimulations.

Endorphins are a natural part of our body's reactions. It's how we normally feel pleasure, like laughing, sexual excitement, eating and exercising. These are wonderful, normal and healthy feelings.

The danger comes with using food as a self-induced pleasure, because endorphins released from eating provide similar effects upon our bodies as those created by narcotic drugs. They cause the body to temporarily feel satisfied, happy, even fulfilled and more relaxed, simply by manipulating the brain's biochemistry. Many foods can cause this reaction but sugar and chocolate are on top of the list and for others it is savory foods.

Interestingly, science shows that when someone is in love their body produces a chemical called phenylethylamine, which as we all know causes us to feel good; it creates a sense of euphoria. Guess what – chocolate contains phenylethylamine and another chemical, theobromine! These chemicals activate endorphins in the brain producing a 'falling in love' feeling. No wonder it's been called 'the love food'.

By eating, or overeating, certain trigger foods a true state of anesthesia can be achieved, dulling the mind or the pain and making the body drowsy. Creating an aura that blocks out the need to cope mentally or emotionally with real life.

Whilst the natural endorphins released after eating can take the edge off the immediate emotional problem, they can also lead to compulsive overeating or dependency. They encourage a false reliance on the body's natural endorphins, a reliance that can only be maintained and satisfied by eating. Sole enjoyment then comes from the pleasure of food, not from life in the now. Over time, this can escalate to addictions, cravings, weight gain and serious health issues.

By its mere existence, comfort eating can lock anyone into an endless cycle of escapism, unfulfilment, depression and overeating. Because food is only a short-term anesthetic it must be eaten more and more frequently to avoid the endorphin level dropping. People are then fooled through habit, to think they are actually hungry, when in reality they aren't physically hungry but emotionally so.

It may have been an external reason that caused the emotional pain, depression, sadness or lack of fulfillment in the first place, but after time it's the above cycle that helps reinforce the negative state. People can easily become emotionally dependent on food to cope with everyday life. I know this is true not only because I see it daily in my clinic but during an extreme stress time in my own life I have found myself in this very situation.

The danger of eating incorrectly and having negative emotions is that they combine to maintain the very symptoms we need to resolve. Why? Because the chemicals that make us think, feel and move (Serotonin, Melatonin, Cortisol and Norepinephrine) are depleted or put out of balance in the brain cells.

When this happens we experience:

- Loss of energy/extreme tiredness
- Weight gain (from overeating)
- Depression/anxiety
- Insomnia
- Accident-prone tendencies
- A feeling of being unloved
- Less motivation
- Anorexia/bulimia
- Hyperactivity
- Lack of concentration
- Stress/anxiety
- Moodiness/melancholy

Understanding this information and the ramifications of it, can surely only lead to the decision to change. A change that can only be brought about by you:

1. Recognizing and understanding your individual situation.
2. Accepting that no food, drug or stimulant can ever fulfill your heart's desires. If you truly want fulfillment, and I know it may seem hard but you will have to change.
3. Realizing you can do something about it.
4. Desiring to do something about it.
5. Actually doing something about it. Take up the challenge. Take your mind off food and put your energies into achieving something else in life. Don't fill the space in your life with another form of escapism, do something progressive and worthwhile. Find something to get your life back in balance.

For example: enroll in a vegetarian cooking class, meet new people, try a new sport, join a gym, put time into old friendships, find a hobby, join in a church group, enroll in study courses, stimulate something in your career, help other people, pursue spiritual fulfillment. The list is endless. Spend time creating a plan and goals. Organize a think-tank and get friends or family to help you with your plan.

Commit to it by writing it down and be answerable to time frames – don't procrastinate.

I encourage you; this is the perfect time. Personal growth is something we all need to work on and the sense of achievement it brings can change your life. It's your decision.

Let this diet be the beginning, the catalyst for you to prosper in emotions, body and spirit. Use it as a partial fast unto God, to get a health breakthrough or healing in your current situation.

This is the time for you to break negative cycles and to move on to something new and exciting in your life - because you deserve to get the best out of life.

What's Your Problem?

Hopefully the revelation of what is being discussed here has forced you to stop and ponder for a moment. This section is not meant to bring up old past hurts just for the sake of it, but to enable reaction patterns and thoughts to be recognized, accepted and understood so that something can be done to improve them.

Sub-conscious thoughts and self-talk like;

"I am overeating because if I'm overweight I don't have to worry about the opposite sex." A lot of people have been abused or hurt in their life by other people, and they reason that by eating and being overweight they are less attractive and therefore safer.

"I am overeating because it helps me cope with the daily stresses and insecurities of life." As I discussed earlier food can tranquillize us. When we become dependent on this food addiction, our ability to cope with the hurdles of life can be hindered greatly.

"Food is a friend, my companion; it's always there for me. It'll never let me down. It'll never reject me." Food is often used to compensate for past rejections and loneliness, to cover the pain, to hide the need to show our true selves and risk being hurt again.

"I am over (or under) eating because it's one thing I have control of in my life." This indicates that the person feels they are not in charge of their decisions, everyday events, their life or even its direction. It can be from having a controlling parent, spouse, or difficult life circumstances. Food intake, in this instance, is seen as one of the few things that the eater can control.

"Food makes life bearable." Childhood pain and past hurts may lead to bingeing. Food can temporarily lessen the pain and block out the memories.

"I have wasted my life. I haven't done any of the things I had wanted to." Frustration and lack of fulfillment with life can lead to obsessive eating habits. A wife may have planned to travel the world; a man may have wanted to turn his hobby into a successful business, you may have been called to do missionary work, but because of whatever reasons (marriage, children, parents, poverty, wrong decisions etc) their dreams remain unfulfilled. So food or drink becomes the tranquillizer to dull the pain and help them forget.

Every individual reacts differently. At this point of the book some readers may be thinking, "I don't come under any of these categories."

But here are a few other mindsets and wrong thinking that can also cause problems.

- "I'm on my own every night; I enjoy/need my food treats. It's my reward and comfort"
- "It's all too hard. I just can't be bothered eating properly."
- "It's my husband's/wife's/kids'/boss'/God's fault."
- "I'm stressed out. Foods help me relax."
- "I'm too busy to prepare meals and eat properly."
- "I just love chocolate, (or cheese, wine, bread, cake, cookies, etc) and I don't want to give it up. So why should I?"
- "I'm a New Testament Christian and free of any Old Testament law, so I can do whatever I want, when I want."
- "I'm believing God for my Healing, so I don't have to change my lifestyle/diet." (Often the lifestyle or diet is the very thing causing the illness in the first place). This is why I continually say "**we all should work with God for our healing, not against Him.**" (More information in FAQ section)

The list of reasons, self justification and excuses can, and does, go on and on and on and on.

But what if none of these excuses are the real reason? What if the real issue is half buried in the past, and digging it up would bring back too many terrible memories? Or perhaps, it's something current that's not only hard to handle, but painful too?

It might seem easier to many just to eat. But, after all that eating, there is often the feeling of guilt from bingeing that has to be faced up to. So another visit is made to the pantry/cookie jar or fridge for more comfort food. And so another step in the vicious and seemingly unending cycle is taken. The result of these steps leads to weight gain, toxic build up and possibly further depression and lethargy and feeling tired all the time. Not to mention disease in the years that follow.

The solution is learning to react differently when your emotional 'buttons' are pushed. It's important to recognize that as everyone is different so are the reasons for reaching for food. Still once the reason for the abnormal hunger is found, the response can be changed and another way can be found to deal with the situation or stress, one that doesn't include heading straight for the cookie jar or wine bottle.

We must be so careful that food doesn't start to be used to meet our emotional, social and spiritual needs.

Change is essential in life. Otherwise, our minds will be leading us around and around the same mountain forever. The pattern has to be broken. Failure to change can lead to yo-yo dieting *(refer to Quick and Healthy Weight Loss section –chapter 5)*, sadness or depression and this is disastrous for the body, mind and spirit.

I have heard nearly all the excuses for not staying on a diet; in fact, I have tried most of them myself. Let's give excuses the boot and become responsible for our own actions and bodies.

Renew Your Mind

"And do not be conformed to this world, but be transformed by the renewing of your mind, that you may prove what is the good and acceptable and perfect will of God." (Romans 12:2).

When dealing with emotional eating, our mind is the source of most of our trouble. The mind is also the area where most battles will be won or lost. Therefore, it stands to reason that we have to think clearly and positively. Negative mindsets and old ways of thinking must be changed.

Why not take some time to recognize and understand what triggers off any emotional responses you might have? It's essential to be honest with yourself. Then, once the trigger is discovered and exposed, keep a record of your responses to this emotional stimulus.

Some examples might be:
> I'm feeling down because I have not received an expected phone call = ice cream and cake.
> My husband never tells me he loves me and he refuses to communicate = chocolate and coffee
> I'm bored = wine, cheese, crackers and/or packet chips
> My boss doesn't appreciate me. I'm overworked = coffee and donuts, later wine and chocolate.
> I'm lonely = a trip to the local Deli for food you know you don't need.
> No one loves me, no one cares how I feel = chocolate and more chocolate...

Case History

Jo, (41 and overweight) had Type 2 diabetes, high blood pressure, fluid retention and was taking anti-depressants.

She completed Daniel's Diet for 10 days and followed a modified Daniel's Diet for a further month, lost 26.5 pounds (12 kg) and was feeling a lot better physically. **However the diet, as it can do, brought to the surface some emotional issues forcing Jo to realize that she was an emotional eater.** *Since she didn't receive any credit or appreciation from her boss or her husband, food had became her self-reward. She was using it as a 'reward system' for her hard work.*

As Jo was telling me this she started crying, and this became the beginning of her healing. She knew it would take time and effort to overcome the habit but together we started forming a plan to break her cycle of reward eating, replacing it with other more positive things, including prayer.

After Jo had worked out how to reward herself differently another problem surfaced. She noticed she would eat junk food when she was annoyed with her husband. Over the years in her marriage she had lost emotional communication with her husband and so she would overeat to spite and rebel against him. Having realized this Jo decided to protect her health and feel better about herself by changing her reactions. It worked.

Once each causative factor is recognized, the first step in winning the battle is taken. The battle, however, is not a skirmish but one that needs fighting all the way to victory. It may not be easy. Professional help may be required. Overcoming self-image problems and wrong or hurtful past experiences is hard but it's necessary for long-term health and healing.

Don't underestimate the power of prayer and faith in the healing process. It has been researched that prayer raises the body's natural immunity quite significantly, as well as forming a link to God. Praying will lift your faith and hope, giving you the strength to do things that perhaps you couldn't before. The Bible teaches us the power of prayer and says that fervent prayer achieves much. (James 5:16)

How to Recognize Emotional Danger Times
Are food cravings worse when you are?
- Watching TV?
- Bored or frustrated?
- Angry or upset with someone?
- Lonely or have a wounded heart?
- Disappointed or unfulfilled with your life?
- Socializing or visiting friends?

Recognizing triggers. Write them down:
- What is the trigger causing you these danger times for you?
- Is it a feeling, habit or memory?
- What is making you see/feel things in a way that causes this reaction?

....

....

....

....

Most people's reactions are due to:
- Life experiences or hurts from the past/present
- Culture, upbringing, environment
- Disappointments
- Abuse – physical, mental or emotional
- Fear of the future/change
- Wrong teachings
- Guilty conscience
- Habits (resistance to change)
- Reactions to, or beliefs in, your perception of truth
- Co-dependency cycles
- Unfulfilled goals or dreams
- Rebellion

Any past experiences can create a thought pattern, or inroad, into the mind. These patterns or paths are imprinted one by one, regardless of whether the pattern is positive or negative, happy or sad, fearful or loving, good or bad. This creates trigger points or buttons that can be pushed by thought or circumstances and when your button has been pushed you will invariably respond the same way every time.

Attitudes and beliefs are formed from past experiences and they are as much a part of us today as they were the day they happened. Just as they affect our responses, so they affect our self-talk. Over time (if not correctly dealt with) these patterns or inroads, become a mental, emotional or spiritual stronghold, and this is where habits are formed.

Realization and understanding are the first steps to overcoming all past or present stimuli. And I believe that once that step is taken, with the help of this book, everyone has the ability to start out on his or her journey towards freedom and success. The teachings in this book have already helped many people to free themselves from ill health, excess weight or emotional pressure as well as offering everyone the opportunity for people to become spiritually awakened and fulfilled.

Why not let it be the beginning or the catalyst for you too?

The Importance of Change

The root of behavioral change is in the subconscious mind, not the conscious. So it's not new thoughts that are required for change, but renewed patterns of thinking – uprooting old, wrong mind patterns, beliefs and reactions to replace them with positive ones. This must be followed by ACTION on your part. Knowledge without action is a non-event.

STEPS of ACTION

Step 1. Read this book. (Be encouraged, this one you've already started).

Step 2. Follow the diet and advice it contains.

Step 3. Recognize and give up all your danger foods.

Step 4. Take up regular exercise.

Step 5. Become a positive thinker and spend time with other positive people.

Step 6. Read more on health.

Step 7. Feed your soul with 'spiritual' food. I believe reading the Bible is the best way to do this.

Step 8. Seek wise council and avoid people who make you feel negative.

Step 9. Find something achievable to accomplish after this diet and work towards a goal.

Step 10. Enjoy the journey.

Most people change some thought patterns occasionally. After attending a seminar, the husband may buy his wife flowers. The wife may make his favorite dinner. However, unless this action continues and progresses into a regular event, it won't become part of the subconscious and therefore, won't be a lasting lifestyle/behavioral change. In other words, actions need to be repeated to become a normal part of you. It has to be a change in the deep mindset to last.

Change is rarely easy. Changing a wife/husband, location, etc. is generally not the answer. The problem is internal, not external, so the change must be internal too. Old thoughts and habits don't get left behind when you move location or change partners. They are taken with you.

A mental, emotional and even spiritual fight might have to be fought and won before the rewards of victory and achievement are realized. And when it's been achieved, the sufferer becomes the victor over the thing or things that were harmful. It's more than an experience or a battle; it's a lifestyle change.

MAJOR OBSTACLES to CHANGE
- Lack of knowledge
- Laziness, slothfulness, lack of discipline
- Hidden or suppressed emotional hurts, frustration and needs
- Cultural mindsets
- Negative self-talk
- Ill health
- Fear
- Lack of good nutrition (creating a lack of mental energy and therefore motivation to make the change)
- Lack of support and understanding from others
- Lack of self worth
- Insecurity and fear
- Stubbornness and rebellious spirit

Changing Self Talk
Do you realize that each one of us talks to our 'self' more in our mind, than to any other person?

So it's vital that this self-talk is positive, uplifting, encouraging and progressive. Listen to what you say to yourself (and to others). The Scriptures say that the power of life and death are in the tongue (proverbs 18:21) and every person's success or failure can hinge on this one point.

Self-talk is all about you, what you think and what is really going on inside you. It has created all your beliefs and feelings, and it controls what you instinctively say and do. It also attracted the situation you find yourself in now.

Self-talk is a major key to achieving goals because it can change your internal programming. It deals directly with the root of the problem or is intimately involved with success. Huge changes, wonderful achievements, success and happiness can all happen in your life simply by changing one or two things in your self-talk.

If you become your own motivator, there's a greater chance of you overcoming problems, staying on a good diet and living a healthy lifestyle. Motivation means to 'put into motion.' Everyone can take control back in his or her life; put their decision to change into motion and follow this healthy way of living.

See yourself slimmer, trimmer and healed of all past issues. Start speaking in a way that encourages you to achieve what you want. Start telling yourself the truth - you are a wonderful, successful person who is going to achieve all they want in life and what's more, you're going to enjoy the journey. The most powerful motivation is your internal motivation. Now is the time to set it into motion!

What If I Don't Change?

Warning - If addiction and unhealthy cycles aren't broken they will lead to an ongoing health problem and a breakdown somewhere in your system. It will appear somewhere in the physical, mental, emotional and may eventually affect the spiritual side of life.

You see, if our inner needs are constantly covered over and continually numbed with momentary pleasure, the problem will never be overcome. Hiding from the cause of the problem actually stops us from finding or reaching what we want so much in our life - consequently we miss out.

For example - Physically if you have a food allergy but keep eating the culprit food then the symptoms you have now will get progressively worse, often appearing in another part of your body manifesting as another health symptom and you end up with a second and even third problem, but all originating in one causative factor. With age, multiple ailments develop and people wonder why.

Since the way we think and speak controls us to such a large degree, I suggest that every reader make a conscious decision saying, "I will take serious notice of the information in this book," "I will change". "It will improve my life."

Re-read the book as many times as you have to, do the diet as many times as you need to, until the results appear. You only have to begin and good things start to happen. Keep working at your success.

Our subconscious doesn't know the truth. It knows only what we program it to believe as truth. That is why we are comfortable with old thought patterns and actions. They are what we know as 'normal,' even if they are self-destructive. Changing these thought patterns and actions will take some effort - but it's possible and it's essential for overall good health.

First, the decision to change: When this choice is made, each altered action will begin to override old behavioral patterns in the control centre of the brain. Eventually the changes will become evident by the internal self-talk then by what is said (or confessed) verbally. Stop and listen to yourself. What are you saying?

There's a speech centre in the brain. It gives anything we say or think direct influence, or controlling power, over most areas of our body. Which means we give negative thoughts control over our body when we repeatedly say or think them.

Negative thoughts like:
- "I'll never lose this weight."
- "I'm tired."
- "I'm lonely."
- "I'm not good enough."
- "God never answers my prayers."
- "Nobody likes me."
- "I can't do this diet."
- "I'm sick."
- "I'm depressed."
- "I'm unlucky."
- "I'll always be fat."
- "I'll never change."
- "I'm fat."
- "I'm too old to change."

These phrases, and others like them, will eventually build-up and have a direct effect upon our emotions, physical body and spirit. One, two or all three of these parts will eventually believe the self-talk and respond accordingly. However, the beauty of this is that when positive thoughts overcome the negative, good things will happen.

Positive thoughts like:
- "I will change my bad habits."
- "God does answer my prayers."
- "I can do all things through Jesus."
- "I love salads and vegetables."
- "I am worthy."
- "Salads are not rabbit food – but Gods creation for me."
- I do enjoy exercise
- "I will lose weight."

Each person's life is a manifestation of what is done or said, in our minds and in our spoken words.

The Power of Your Words
I believe this whole section holds a major key to why some people do, and some people don't, overcome short and long-term problems. Try using the theory of positive thought in any area of life. Just try it. When used correctly and consistently, I have no doubt that the success you desire will be achieved.

Case History
Linda, (41 years) had successfully completed Daniel's Diet and was six months into her moderation diet. She had already achieved her goal weight.

Linda had tried various diets before but could never stay on any of them for long. She gave her testimony in my teaching class.

"What made the difference," she said, "was that I changed my self talk from negative to positive. I was always saying to myself and to my friend's negative things

about my body shape and weight problem. Discussing my weight, how hard diets were and my health issues became a social conversation topic. My friends would all agree with me and I with them and I wondered why I was stuck in a rut and couldn't get out. Then we would end the pity party by indulging in coffee with milk and sugar followed with cookies and cakes."

Changing:

- *"First my group of friends, until I was strong enough not to be influenced by them."*
- *"Then my self talk and confession of what I spoke."*
- *"This diet is too hard."*
- *"I hate this food."*
- *"My bottom is too big"*
- *"I look fat."*
- *"Nothing will ever make me feel/look better."*

To:

- *"I love my new lifestyle."*
- *"I love natural foods."*
- *"I am working with God not against Him."*
- *"I look and feel great."*
- *"I like who I am."*
- *"I love my bottom."*
- *"I want to be healthy for me, my family and God."*
- *"God loves me."*

Linda used these positive affirmations long enough for them to become her normal response and belief. She overrode her old destructive thought patterns and won the battle over negative self-talk.

What are your negative affirmations (thoughts and words)?

1..

2..

3..

4..

5..

Change them from negative to positive.

1..

2..

3..

4..

5..

Having written your negative thoughts down to identify them, now never use them again. Use the positive ones instead. It only takes thirty days of conscious positive self-talk to beat past habits and to make the change.

Understanding The Body's Responses To Emotional Triggers.
The human body has no nature of its own. It will do whatever it's told to do. Tell yourself to stand, sit, go to the bathroom, lift your arm over your head or eat some ice cream. You see what I mean? The human body will do whatever we tell or train it to do.

Our physical bodies are programmed to such a degree that they will function automatically, without conscious direction. We can walk, talk, eat, breathe or drive a car with little, or no, conscious thought. The commands we give could be good or bad, negative or positive, but our bodies will still do them.

There is no question about it – we can each reprogram ourselves. If our thoughts determine our behaviour and our actions, then they also have a huge influence on our emotions.

I myself have been conditioned from childhood to have food responses. I used to come home from school, and find comfort by eating half a packet of biscuits (cookies). To this day after a hard day's work when I come home and need to relax, what happens? My conditioned response kicks in. I find myself having to resist the urge to eat something sweet, because of this I endeavor to have fruit or something healthy on hand: nuts and sun-dried fruit or unsweetened carob with ginger, for example. I also find having a high density Protein shake (I use ones made from Pea or Brown Rice. See more in Q&A section) helps stop the cravings, when used at the appropriate times. Don't let food or emotions control you. You can control them.

I believe emotional eating is the biggest hurdle to overcome in losing weight especially over long term and controlling food addictions and the co dependency on food!

By reaching this stage of realization and understanding, a healthy lifestyle (including your perfect weight) becomes much easier to maintain; success is yours to enjoy.

I often counsel people who say they have to eat a cookie or a slice of cake every time they have a cup of tea or coffee. Why do they feel this way? Once again, it's a conditioned response. And it's a way of thinking that can only be broken by understanding the body's response and changing it.

In the above situation, the cup of tea or coffee triggers the craving for sweetness. Therefore, a simple solution to avoid this craving is to stop having the hot drink. No coffee = no urge for cookies or cake. It's an easy solution, resulting in a positive change in the patient's weight and health. Stop or avoid anything that feeds the cravings or habit. If it's a

TV advert showing you how enticing ice cream is – swap channels while it's on, don't feed the cravings in your mind.

Sometimes life can seem empty, lonely, unfulfilled, and loveless. If it is, succumbing to destructive habits and negative self-talk can become all too easy. But if people start to fill their lives with these destructive things it's going to lead to bigger problems. The longer artificial and synthetic supports, like food, alcohol, excess TV, medications and other drugs, are depended upon, the harder it becomes to break the cycle. Under the pressure of stress or emotional pain, a night or two of eating ice cream, chips or chocolate is understandable, most of us have done that at some time. However, it's dangerous when a month goes by and the comfort food is still being eaten each night. It's becoming a habit.

Alcohol, drugs, excess TV and DVDs, excess sports or becoming a workaholic are all possible addictions/escapisms that can become un-natural supports.

If you see any of these traits in your character please, for your own sake and for those around you, acknowledge your reactions to different stresses and emotional circumstances and CHANGE.

In order to overcome a dependency, it's vital to face up to any emotional control or reaction that is ruling your body and mind. If inner needs are not being met, physically, emotionally, mentally or spiritually, that is when comfort food can become a dependency. At the time it may appear to be the answer. But it's a false answer. It offers a temporary solution and won't meet your long-term needs. There may be momentary gratification but it doesn't come close to meeting the real needs. It's not even a stopgap. It's actually less than a stopgap measure, because it helps to hide the true need and leads away from fulfillment. Remember, if these needs are not faced up to, habits intensify and the vicious cycle continues - a cycle that worsens with every rotation, stealing peace and health as it goes.

Thought patterns and past conditioning, along with taste buds, will change. Weight can be lost and kept off. We can all overcome and find health, vitality and peace in life.

Stop the Old 'Stinking Thinking'

YOU CAN DO IT! It's crucial to discover your foremost times of temptation. That way you can choose to do something different at that time. For many it's around four or five o'clock in the afternoon when our blood sugar is low and the need to have a healthy snack is strong. For others it's in the evenings, after dinner while relaxing or watching TV.

Try to replace bad, old habits with:

- Exercising.
- Eating healthy snacks - eat a healthy snack before temptation hits.
- Helping people - helping others distracts us all from our own problems. Turn outwards in your thinking, instead of inwards, and give a helping hand to others.
- Prayer and reading the Bible - both have given comfort to countless people, including myself. It's also a powerful way to find answers for your personal situation.
- Meeting new friends - maybe join a church group or a charity organization.
- Mixing with people who are positive, encouraging and happy.
- Creative activity - enjoying and accomplishing things is always a great help. Try something that is ongoing and gives a sense of achievement.
- Being content with your life - even if you desire things to be different in the future, be happy with what you have now. Plan for the future and enjoy the journey.

Responsibility

Our health is a gift from God and we have to look after and nourish it. Never take it for granted.

No matter how we look at this, none of us can escape the responsibility of managing our own body. Nobody else can do it for us, nobody should be expected to. Health does not occur through luck or chance.

We have to make the choices that are right for us. It's our job to maintain the engine by providing it with the right fuels. It's something we can all do.

Be Aware Of What Your Body Is Telling You

To determine which foods are causing you to be tired, depressed or lethargic, monitor how you feel after you've eaten. Do you feel tired, unable to concentrate, have stomach bloating or pain, maybe feel depressed or irritable? Be aware of whether you are hypersensitive, allergic or intolerant to a certain food or substance. If you're not sure of your reactions write down everything you eat over a one - two week period.

First, you write down breakfast, mid morning, lunch, afternoon, dinner, snacks, drinks etc. note what foods are being listed daily or nearly every day. It may be the same cereal or bread every morning, the same bread roll for lunch, the same sweets or deserts every evening.

I know that after eating oat meal with milk for breakfast, within thirty to sixty minutes I feel mentally tired and struggle to concentrate. The same reaction happens with sugar and packet cereals, this indicates I'm sensitive to grains and sugar.

After a large lunch many people just want to lie down and have a siesta, this can be from sensitivities to what you ate or from an overload on your digestion.

Next, write down how you feel emotionally and physically in the time from consuming that food or drink until the next time you eat or drink. Reactions or signs can be between five minutes or three to four hours, after eating. This way it may be possible to see a pattern emerging and this will tell you what's triggering different responses.

Be your own food and emotions detective. See the common denominator to the foods that make you feel any unnatural sensations. Usually it's substances like bread, cereal, packet foods, instant noodles, junk food, sugar, cheese, milk, etc. However, it can be any food or drink and be aware that it can also be multiple substances or combinations that cause symptoms. One of my favorite sayings is, "be in tune with your body –

symptoms are warning signs and you have to listen to them."

Case History

Jan, (mid 20's and a TV personality) originally consulted with me because she was in desperate need of help. Jan's symptoms were multiple and getting worse with time.

They were: chronic tiredness, poor concentration, lethargy, headaches, back pain, menstrual problems, mood swings (emotional highs and lows) and she was also unable to fall pregnant.

Jan loved her job, but her concentration span was becoming very limited and it was becoming increasingly difficult for her to handle the pressure. All Jan's symptoms and resultant tiredness and unhappiness were becoming too much for her. At this stage of her life she was seriously considering quitting work and leaving her husband. In fact, even her life was becoming too much for her.

It was very evident in my consult with Jan that she had, over time, developed very poor eating and lifestyle habits. Jan was literally existing from day to day by propping herself up with artificial stimulation from food and drink.

Jan's eating habits were:

Breakfast - a cigarette and a coffee, with milk and two sugars.

Mid-morning - coffee, cigarette, a dry wheat cracker with margarine and a yeast-based spread followed by a cake or cookies.

Lunch - a salad sandwich with ham or cheese, orange juice and a chocolate candy bar. Or sometimes she had a savory meat pie with tomato ketchup.

Afternoon Tea – cookies or chocolate and an occasional piece of fruit, always with coffee.

Dinner (always 9.00 pm or later) - consisted of: meat, chicken or curry and white rice, casserole or pasta, each with the same two or three vegetables and dessert. Followed by several coffees and chocolate, occasionally with alcohol as well.

Jan's other eating habits included take-out chicken, or hamburger and fries, three or four times a week. She was also drinking twelve cups/mugs of coffee a day, as well as two or three cans of caffeinated soda.

Exercise

Jan had stopped all forms of exercise and now did not have the energy to undertake any new programs.

Sleep - Jan slept six hours each night.

Jan's first attempt to take up Daniel's Diet failed.

I had explained the life changes, vitamins/herbs and Daniel's Diet to Jan at the first consultation. But after a brief attempt, Jan rang me and opted out of the program. It seemed too hard for her to give up all her 'goodies'.

It isn't easy to change when there are so many problem foods. Giving up sugar or chocolate can be as hard as giving up cigarettes or alcohol and Jan was a chocoholic as well as being addicted to the others foods.

However, three months later she came back to see me, even more desperate than before. Jan explained that it had taken a severe fluctuation in her health and the near collapse of her marriage before she and her husband made the mental decision to get my help. In fact, it was an act of sheer desperation. Their marriage was on the edge of divorce.

This time, Jan followed the program in stages, giving up her addictions one at a time. First went the chocolate and sugars, next the coffee and junk food, then finally cigarettes. All this took only two months by which time she was feeling better and better with each passing week, which encouraged her to keep going with her lifestyle changes.

Jan was now ready to do Daniel's Diet and when she had completed the 10 days the results were staggering.

The Results

Within two weeks of finishing the diet and two and a half months from the commencement of the plan, there was no further need for a psychologist or marriage guidance counselor. In fact, Jan's husband was so impressed with her progress and change of temperament that he'd volunteered to follow her lifestyle changes. The two of them were astounded at the improvements in their personal moods, general health and energy levels.

Jan stated, "It's unbelievable. I am not moody or irritable any more. We've both changed, we're a lot calmer and relaxed, and we hardly ever fight." About the initial withdrawal stages she said, "It was hard, but I knew I had to weather the storm. Having a program to follow and knowing it was worth the effort gave us the strength to continue. It's amazing the difference I feel just through diet and lifestyle changes."

Conclusion

The latest report on Jan and her husband one year on is that she is still working on TV and loving it. Her energy and concentration are great. She is very happy in her marriage. She's pregnant with their first child (remember she couldn't fall pregnant before) and finishing a degree that she had previously abandoned because of her lack of energy and concentration. Jan is also going back to her church and has recommitted her life to God.

I know these tools will help, so open your spiritual toolbox and use them!

CHAPTER SEVEN

CRAVINGS AND ADDICTIONS

An addiction to food can be very intense. It can have a hold on a person that is just as strong as an addiction to cigarettes and alcohol. Overeating is often wrongly justified, considered morally or socially more acceptable unlike smoking and drunkenness. It shouldn't be. They are all life threatening.

Recognize the Enemy

The emotional cravings I have discussed under, 'Are You an Emotional Eater?' deals with the internal addiction. The main physical trigger that causes a craving is an internal chemical and toxic irritation of the tissue and nervous system.

This is usually brought about by:

- Over-consumption of irritant foods e.g. wheat, sugar or refined foods
- Chemicals added to food
- Soils being sprayed with toxic chemicals
- Mineral deficient foods (because of deficient soils)

The first step to overcoming this type of addiction is to recognize and understand that it exists. Face the facts. Many people don't understand this connection to their health, whilst others are in denial about their addictive eating habits and the link between the food and their emotions. Some are even in denial about the possible health consequences until something serious happens. But why wait until you are dangerously ill before doing anything about it?

How Man-Made Chemicals React Within Us

Most people eat processed foods daily, but our bodies were just not made to handle the thousands of man-made chemicals that these foods contain. Each year, literally thousands of new chemical food additives, most of which are foreign to our systems, are produced. Admittedly, not all are harmful, but many are.

These chemicals can cause an irritation in our nervous system that travels right through our body down to the gut. This reaction, day in day out, eventually demands to be soothed, and because eating more of the substance (that originally caused the irritation) gives immediate relief, the body sends out messages requesting more of that food

However, this solution only works in the short term. Eventually the irritation and craving starts up again and we, misreading the signal, hunt out and consume more of the detrimental substance, or one from the same family. Here is where the vicious cycle is established.

Highly refined carbohydrates, such as sugar, white rice, and white flour based products, cereals and most bread can abnormally stimulate the intestinal tract into triggering a secretion called Neuro Hormone. This hormone establishes a physical dependency on these antagonistic substances.

Eating the craved substance will seem to sooth the internal irritation and immediately satisfy, but its consumption will inadvertently create not just obesity but a huge myriad of bad health symptoms too.

This scenario often leads to a lifestyle of yo-yo dieting, guilt and never being able to stay on any diet for long. It can create a situation where we find ourselves eating certain foods, even though we know we shouldn't. Negative thoughts and self-talk might follow, to the extent where people just give up on a healthy diet because it seems all too hard. Or perhaps drug therapy becomes more appealing, in the hope that a new 'instant weight-loss pill' will miraculously create the perfect slim body without the work.

If entrenched long enough, the chemical imbalance, caused by food addiction, may alter normal thought processes by confusing nerve impulses. This makes it more and more difficult for the mind to comprehend and believe what is happening. At this stage, the dependency reaches a point where the brain will stop any possible thought that the addictive food is bad. This is denial.

Self-justification and excuses seem like the truth. Justifications like:
- "Why should I eat healthy food?"
- "It's too hard; I like these foods, why should I give them up?"
- "I can lose weight anytime I want to. I just don't want to diet now."
- "I'll go on the diet next week or maybe next month"
- "It's my metabolism. It's slow; I was born with it that way, so I can never lose weight."
- "It doesn't matter what I look like, people love me because of who I am inside."
- "I'm not getting much love and attention but what's that got to do with my obesity and sweet tooth?"
- These common statements are indicative of being controlled and hooked on food substances.

How to check yourself for food sensitivities or allergies
- Create a Food Diary over seven days; write down everything you consume. For example:
    * Breakfast - cereal with milk and sugar, cup of coffee with milk and sugar…etc
    * Morning Snack - two choc-chip cookies, cup of tea or coffee with milk
    * Lunch Sandwich with…
    * Afternoon…
    * Dinner…
    * And so on.
- What are the foods that keep regularly appearing in your diet?

- Which food or drink show up daily, or nearly every day?

Compare your list of regularly eaten foods with the one below. Over my twenty years of diet analysis the most common culprits I see listed are:

- milk/cheese
- cereals
- pasta
- chocolate
- sodas
- alcohol
- candy/sweets
- pastry foods
- Pizza
- pies/pasties
- pudding/sweets

- bread
- caffeine
- white rice
- ice cream
- flavored milks
- cookies and savory biscuits/crackers
- Chinese take-out
- instant noodles
- orange juice
- instant noodles
- Take out e.g. Hamburgers (fries), soda, fried fish & chips

Can you see any similarities between the lists? Now is the time to admit to your most repeated and possibly addictive foods.

Confession time

One of the best ways to be sure that you are being honest and free of denial is to talk to a friend or family member. To verbally state you have a food addiction is to fully acknowledge it. I also suggest writing it down for your own accountability.

Now that the possible addictions have been acknowledged it's time to do something about them.

For accuracy it's probably best to select no more than one or two foods/drinks at a time.

Now go off the chosen food(s) you have named for seven days.

Record what happens – your body will tell you.

- Which food do you really miss, crave and think about?

- In the seven days did you get a headache?
- Did you feel weak, listless and perhaps even get the shakes?
- Were you moody or irritable?
- Did you recognize any withdrawal signs?
- Was your mind rebelling against the whole idea?

If it's extremely hard to stop eating certain foods in order to follow this diet then be encouraged, you're not the only one. It isn't always easy to stop eating addictive foods but now is the time to recognize and break their hold on you. Completing this diet is the key.

Case History

Joy heard me give a talk on physical food addictions. The information was a revelation to her and she checked her normal food intake in the way I just mentioned. After doing the food checks she couldn't believe the withdrawal symptoms she had from certain foods. Joy was so shocked by what her body was showing her that she changed her lifestyle immediately, all her negative health symptoms then disappeared.

After attending just two lecture meetings, Joy said, "I don't have to come back any more because I have changed my lifestyle, I'm now eating only the foods from God's Garden and doing just fine."

Joy had:

1. *Heard (a lack of knowledge was no longer an excuse)*
2. *Made a decision (purposed in her mind)*
3. *Acted on her decision (became a 'doer' of what she had learned)*
4. *Was reaping the benefits (rewards come after action and change)*

I'm sorry but there are no instant, miracle cures for weight-loss. But there are well-balanced weight loss diets like *Daniel's Diet* that can, if followed correctly, be the answer.

There are also powerful herbs that can assist your situation and together with the diet and lifestyle changes you can achieve your ideal weight and health goals.

No one has to battle everything with only their own strength and mind. You are not on your own, there is help and there is a solution to your problem. Natural medicine is there to help.

Personal Strategies That Can Help You Resist Cravings
- Make a plan and commit to it. This book and my other teachings should help set the plan – but you have to carry it out.
- Keep a diary of your daily eating habits and at the end of each week study it and see the common traps and warnings.
- Eat five times a day (as necessary). As long as it's the right food it won't make you put on weight. Don't eat after 7 pm.
- Drink water with a squeeze of lemon juice ($\frac{1}{2}$ lemon) in it to help fight cravings. Also drink fennel tea and eat fennel seeds.
- Keep your mind occupied. Plan ahead and be ready with something fun to fill those times when the thoughts of food swamp your mind.
- Buddy systems: Find a friend or a group who will encourage and help you stay committed and focused on succeeding. You don't have to be perfect, just work on progressing towards your goal. We can all have a bad day or two, but by focusing on the next day, rather than the last, it is easier to get back to the healthy lifestyle that will provide more and more good days.
- I have many patients who find it beneficial to consult with me once a fortnight, or each month. They just need to be accountable for themselves and talk about their good and bad days. These patients find this invaluable in helping them stay on their lifestyle plan. For those who can afford the luxury, having a naturopath and /or a personal trainer is very beneficial.
- The minerals, Chromium, Magnesium, B12, B6 and Iron and the herb, Gymnema, can be priceless in overcoming cravings.

** Go to my web site and I will analyze your diet for you. www.wisdomforhealth.com

Case History

Nova, (22) is an ex-chocoholic (she 'needed' to eat chocolate every day) and a self-confessed carbohydrate craver. She also noticed an uncontrollable increase of cravings the week before and during her menstruation.

"This combination of supplements (Chromium, Magnesium, B12, B6, Iron and Gymnema is the best kept secret in health care," she said. "Everyone should know about it. I never thought I could stop the food cravings but after taking these supplements I no longer have cravings for any of them. Simply amazing."

Menstrual Cravings

Women who suffer this type of craving will know what I mean. It's a craving, around the time of menstruation, for certain foods (usually detrimental ones) like candy, sweets, chocolate, cheese, chips, crackers, etc. It's often caused by a mineral deficiency within the individual and/or hypoglycemia. The deficiency creates the cravings to alert the body of the imbalance so that the missing source of energy can be replaced.

To overcome the cravings I recommend a vitamin supplement containing:
- *Iron*
- *Magnesium*
- *B vitamins*
- *Folic acid*
- *Chromium*
- *Vitamin C*

The formula will need to be taken continuously over several months to feel the full benefits from it. The above combinations can be found in one or maybe two formulas. Seek professional advice to see if you need these nutrients.

CHAPTER EIGHT

BALANCING YOUR BRAIN'S BIOCHEMISTRY

Our greatest asset is our mind. It's linked to our emotions, it's the gateway to our spirit and, at the centre of it, is our brain.

Just as we can care for, strengthen, enhance and repair our bodies, so too can we care for, strengthen, enhance and repair our brain. It functions on a delicate electrochemical balance. And these functions depend entirely on the nutrition we eat. Nutrition is its fuel.

What we eat determines whether it runs properly or not.

If that fuel is dirty (filled with toxins) or of poor quality (lacking nutrition), it will cause disruption of the brain signals and normal functions. The result is a multitude of problems and abnormal brain reactions. These problems affect not only our physical body and mind, but also our emotions, attitudes and even our personalities.

So our brainpower is directly influenced by our daily nutrition. Without even realizing it, many people may be influencing the way they think, behave, act and perceive things, purely by what they choose to eat or not eat.

How the Brain Works

Our brains contain over ten billion nerve cells called 'neurons.' Neurons have countless root-like fibers, each one with a bulb at the end. Out of these bulbs shoot tiny amounts of natural chemicals, which strike the walls of other brain cells with electrical charges.

Each of these charges results in our brain cells releasing other important chemicals. This is happening continuously, millions of times every minute. The chemicals released are called 'neurotransmitters' and our memory, moods, sleep patterns, appetite, attitudes, sex drive and our ability to learn, are all controlled by these neurotransmitters. This process, therefore, has enormous ramifications on everyday behaviour, how we feel, act, think, concentrate and how intellectually focused we are and so on.

Our brain responses are a manifestation of our very personality and since our brains never stop they eat up huge amounts of energy.

Brains need 20% of the total blood pumped from the heart and 25% of the body's oxygen supply. Thirty million conductors, or nerve fibers, transmit information between the two halves of the brain. The energy generated is so powerful it can be measured on an electrical machine (EEG). The brain can send a nerve command to the toes at over 300 km per hour. The brain is so intricate, powerful and complicated that the best intellectual minds of today can't explain its full function.

This whole powerhouse runs on pure fuel and it has to be maintained every day or a malfunction may occur. Can you imagine flying in an airplane when an incorrect or polluted fuel had been put into the jet engines? Well your brain is more intricate, delicate and sensitive than that plane. It's vital to give it the right fuel.

Brain Fuel

Vitamins, minerals, amino acids, glucose and enzymes are the necessary ingredients to keep this awesomely complex organ functioning properly.

What we do, and do not eat, is vital. It is the key to health and maintaining proper bodily function. The correct process is that we eat the right foods, digest them properly and assimilate the nutrients they contain. The nutrients then travel from the gut through the blood into the brain. In this form the brain is able to collect what it needs for its optimal function, the blood is then recycled back to the liver for replenishment and filtering.

Our body breaks down food into individual nutrients and these are then synthesized into pure fuel. If a jet engine, or your car for that matter, is filled up with impure fuel it gets sluggish and eventually stops. So do we! If we aren't eating correctly, we deprive our bodies of one or more of the essential ingredients. It only takes one missing nutrient to cause a malfunction and to dramatically alter nerve cell function, effecting moods, appetite, energy, coordination and behaviour.

If you're experiencing mood swings, energy fluctuations, memory loss, lack of motivation, excessive anger, depression, eye weakness, mental tiredness or lack of concentration, check what you're eating and drinking. It may be having a direct chemical effect on how you feel.

Depression and the Nutritional Link

An unsuspected nutritional deficiency or food allergy may, directly or indirectly, be the primary cause of many emotional problems. The foods we eat are a basic factor in determining our emotional responses or moods. Cravings may well be our body's desperate attempt to regulate its brain chemistry. If the brain is lacking in certain minerals or amino acids it will give you signals, and craving certain foods may be just that signal.

The key is to replenish with the right foods, otherwise it leads to craving of instant gratification foods like sugar and fat, which may appear to help in the short term but makes things worse in the long term.

Food sensitivities or allergies can cause extreme negative reactions in so-called 'normal' people.

Manifestations may include:

- Anger
- Crying
- Withdrawal
- Memory loss
- Brain fatigue
- Tiredness
- Depression
- Introvert behavior
- Poor concentration

Case Study

Sam (a young lady in her 20's) couldn't believe how she used to cry at the drop of a hat one minute and explode in a fury the next. She had been blaming PMS (pre menstrual syndrome), knowing that sometimes it could be the cause but she was growing increasingly unsure of whether it really was, due to the frequency and timing of her emotional outbursts.

Sam explained that recently whilst on a wonderfully romantic evening with her boyfriend, she had drunk a couple of glasses of wine. Then on the drive home, after eating a packet of potato chips, the whole feeling of the evening had changed and within minutes they were in a totally illogical, raging argument.

Together we tracked her reactions down to intolerance to the additives in potato chips and alcohol. Immediately the culprits had been identified they were omitted from her diet. (She also suffered from Candida Albicans, a yeast infection, which made these reactions to alcohol especially, more enhanced.)

Later, as part of a clinically induced demonstration, the foods were reintroduced and she was amazed at the strength of the now obvious reactions. The dietary changes and introduction of supplements dramatically changed her emotional idiosyncrasies.

As you can appreciate balancing the brain's normal chemicals is of great importance to balancing the body's general well being. Following the diet and lifestyle plan laid out in this book, whilst including supplements, will help produce this balance. But in some advanced cases, a personal evaluation from a practitioner or counselor may be necessary.

What Stops The Brain Working Properly?

- Lack of nutrients
- Lack of water
- Sugar
- Stress
- Lack of sleep
- Junk food
- Alcohol
- Allergies/food sensitivity
- Chemical toxins (including medications and drugs)
- Heavy/toxic metals (lead, mercury, aluminum, cadmium, arsenic, uranium)

Another reason is lack of oxygen. In order for oxygen to be carried to the brain, it needs exercise, correct breathing, enough water and the right minerals.

Summary: To get the maximum out of your brainpower, to balance its biochemistry and to get optimum health, follow this detox program and all the guidelines set out in this book. Keep exercising and challenging your imagination and brain, no matter what your age.

Herbs to help

Herbs to improve your memory, mental performance, concentration and learning abilities include:

1. Bacopa (monniera) also known as Brahmi.
2. Siberian Ginseng
3. Gingko Biloba

These herbs are very helpful in easing mental tiredness (great for students studying), stress and exhaustion and recovery from nervous breakdown; together with Withania and Rhodiola they are truly God's Medicine for today.

Case History

JJ, (a teenage boy) was brought into my clinic by his mum, during the first term of the school year. He was attending boarding school and the teachers were running out of ways to try and help him. JJ's grades were averaging around 25-30%. He couldn't write straight on lined paper, his jumbled words running up and down the page. He struggled to read because even typed words often appeared jumbled and confusing to him.

As we talked, he confessed that in class he found it almost impossible to read off a dry-erase marker board because

Often the words appeared jumbled. He felt so ashamed and bewildered by this that he hadn't told anyone. It was these same reasons that had stopped him telling anyone about the black spots that he saw floating in front of his eyes.

JJ's behavior was erratic. Sometimes he was withdrawn and lethargic, yet at other times he was defensive and rebellious. Immediately we devised and implemented a dietary programme to help him overcome his challenges.

I saw him again halfway through the second of the school's four terms. By the mid-year exams he had progressed from getting a 25% average to getting a 50% average and his whole behavior and personality was beginning to change.

When I saw him at the end of the year his grades were averaging 60%. The floating spots had disappeared. He could write along the lines in textbooks and follow what was on the board, and he could concentrate for much longer. The teachers were amazed by the changes and wanted to know what had been done to get such results.

JJ's mother was overwhelmed and delighted. She brought me letters written to her by her son, each growing in legibility. They also showed his growing ability to express himself normally.

Conclusion

JJ wrote me a lovely poem at the end of the third term (which I still have) showing me just how much this young man had progressed. For years after he would call in to my clinic on his Christmas vacation and chat for a little while, telling me of his progress. He eventually went on to college and become a successful young man. The changes in JJ over the years in mind, body and spirit were truly amazing.

How to Maximize Your Brain Function

Simple, we detoxified JJ's brain and enhanced his blood/brain chemistry with the necessary nutrients. The central nervous system is extremely sensitive to toxins in the blood. By changing his diet and giving JJ the supplements he needed, his body was able to correct itself and function properly. Once the signals sent by his brain were un-jumbled and became normal, his body was able to adjust and heal itself.

It concerns me greatly the number of people whose lives are negatively affected by unrecognized deficiencies and toxic overload. How many young people are struggling at school or work? How many more are quitting school? How many are underachieving, rebelling or have anti-social behaviour because of their diet? Many people do not realize the connection between food (consumables) and behaviour so find it easier to blame something else or just battle on with life. Others feel embarrassed or confused and don't want to talk about the symptoms.

Yet others go to seek professional help and get a wrong diagnosis and are put on treatments that send them off on a tangent and further away from the cause.

They are in essence, borderline ADD or ADHD but are not diagnosed or treated appropriately. Indeed, if JJ had not received the natural treatment he needed he would probably have ended up on medication, under psychiatric treatments or in prison. Instead he got a degree, and is now living a well-balanced, successful life. The same can be said for the executive business person or truck driver. No matter your age, weight or vocation, a detox and an improvement in lifestyle would be a wise investment to your present and future health.

I have lost count of the people who have commented on how much better their concentration and mental stamina is after completing this 10 day Biblical Diet.

CHAPTER NINE

EXPOSING HARMFUL FOODS

Chocolate

- Is chocolate one of your favorite treats?
- Do you eat chocolate daily, or every other day?
- Do you crave chocolate if you don't eat any?
- Are you a chocoholic, a self-confessed lover of this sweet, sticky, gooey bundle of fat, sugar and chemicals?

This strong desire for chocolate is very common and often considered normal. Many people self-justify its consumption because of the momentary enjoyment and the subtle 'high' eating it gives. However, there is a much larger and insidious picture involved than that. This strong desire or need for chocolate is really no more than an addiction or allergy craving.

It's not JUST the soft, sweet, creamy texture that is desired – it's all the other things found in chocolate as well.

Chocolate contains:
1. Fat
2. Sugar
3. Caffeine
4. Chemicals (a. Phenylethylamine b. Theobromine)

These last two chemical substances increase the cravings already triggered by the other ingredients. Both phenylethylamine and theobromine can be addictive, just like the caffeine, sugar and even the fat.

These chemicals actually stimulate the central nervous system. They provide the feeling of energy and give the well-known lift that goes with satisfying a chocolate craving. This lift is just like any other addictive 'kick,' be it alcohol, cigarettes or drugs.

And just like them, when the substance is absorbed and metabolized by the body, it is often followed by a letdown or 'downer' that is only reversed by another dose.

It amazes me the amount of chocolate some people eat, and don't realize the bad side effects on their health and addiction of it. An elderly lady recently consulted with me and she confessed to eating a whole family size chocolate every day and had done so for many years and she wondered why she had developed a series of ill health related issues. Reading this book changed her life and quite probably added years to it.

This Is an Addictive Cycle

Ounce for ounce, pound for pound, chocolate is arguably the most potent mixture of dangerous foods for weight gain and negative health symptoms.

Chocolate - Rat Droppings & Cockroach Body Parts!

Chocolate is made from the cocoa bean which grows on cocoa trees in tropical countries. To combat the many fungi and insects native to these warm and humid regions, pesticides and fungicides are sprayed on the trees, sadly it isn't known how much of these chemicals permeate the actual beans. When harvested, the cocoa beans are left to dry on the ground.

During this time insects and small animals live and feed among the beans, leaving droppings, hairs and dead insects behind them when they go.

After about a week, the beans are packed into bags and stored in warehouses till its time for them to be shipped. Here again rodents and insects contaminate the harvest.

When the bags arrive at the chocolate processing plants, a genuine effort is made to remove as many of these contaminants as possible. But the question is, how do you separate out all these tiny fragments from the tons and tons of cocoa beans? Governments do have regulations to cover this: If 3.5 ounces (100 grams) of chocolate exceeds 60 microscopic insect fragments or one rodent hair, when six samples are analyzed, or if any one sample has more than 90 insect fragments or three rodent hairs, this sample is rejected. However, this means if 3.5 ounces of chocolate has: 60 insect parts OR 1 rodent hair it is considered safe for human consumption.

Despite the possible animal content chocolate carries no disease because all micro-organisms are destroyed in the high temperatures used for processing. Which is good news, but even so the information on harvesting and storing gives food for thought, doesn't it?

Case Study

As a guest speaker one night in Perth, Western Australia, I was relating the story of how chocolate is made when, unbeknown to me, a student on her way to an evening class paused by the door to listen. A few months later she made a point of contacting me.

She told me that for months she had wanted to give up chocolate but had never found the conviction to do it. But since hearing me speak on the amount of rodent hairs, droppings and cockroach parts in chocolate, her interest in the food had been totally destroyed. The information she had received from those few minutes in the doorway had liberated her entirely from the addiction, enabling her to lose weight.

I have repeated the chocolate story (unknown source) many times in talks and discussions, and the above reaction is the reason I tell it so often –even if its tongue in cheek - whatever it takes to break an addiction and help people.

Chocolate and Calcium Deficiency

Both chocolate and cocoa contain a high amount of Oxalic Acid. This acid prevents calcium from being absorbed by the human body. Even the calcium in foods already in the digestive tract cannot be assimilated properly if it comes into contact with the acid.

Since chocolate nearly always comes mixed with sugar, regular consumers can suffer from a variety of problems, regardless of whether they eat chocolate coated candy bars, flavored milks, desserts or any of the many preparations.

Symptoms include:

• Teeth problems	• Nervousness	• Depression
• Heart problems	• Soft bones	• Skin itch

Lastly, osteoporosis sufferers and those who wish to avoid contributing to the development of the disease will benefit greatly from avoiding or reducing this food, along with soda drinks.

Migraine Sufferers

Research shows that at least two thirds of migraines are caused by allergic reactions to foods. Chocolate and dairy foods being high on the list.

I have seen many people who suffer from all types of headaches, never have one again after following Daniel's Diet. I have also seen people who openly admit that their headaches returned when they went back to their old eating habits. This of course is clear proof that diet and headaches are related.

In some stubborn cases enemas or laxatives are needed to help detox the bowel and rid the body of the accumulated toxins, which are causing the headache.

I suggest that those suffering from headaches take the time to wean themselves off chocolate, caffeine, sugar, orange juice and other toxins before starting Daniel's Diet.

Following the plan in the Pre-Diet chapter is recommended and will lessen the withdrawal pain. It's less traumatic on the body to cut out one or two addictive substances at a time, before stopping all together. However, the decision is entirely dependent on the person, their situation, their personality and their determination.

Case Study

An ex SAS soldier heard my lecture on addiction, and said 'I have been praying for

God to take away my headaches for years and finally I know what His answer to me is.' He immediately went on Daniel's Diet. He went from consuming copious amounts of caffeine, milk and sugar, and chocolate to 'cold turkey.'

His comment was, "I had prayer to support me, and what was four days of withdrawal headaches compared to years of recurring headaches. Especially, since after those four days I never suffered another headache again." 'My prayers were answered, but it took a long time for me to listen and obey.'

Chocolate and Menstruation Cravings

I have lost count of the women who have said to me, "I just have to eat chocolate around the time of my period."

Let me tell you, cravings for chocolate at period times of the month are very common.

A strong desire for chocolate is often linked to a mineral deficiency of:

- Iron
- Chromium
- Magnesium
- Zinc

I have witnessed great results with patients overcoming their cravings whilst on Daniel's Diet. They report that after completing the diet and continuing on with the supplements for a further few months their cravings diminish enormously, making the desire easy to overcome. It's important to understand that supplementation is not an overnight solution; supplements must be taken long enough and in the right doses to rectify the deficiencies.

Chocolate and Weight Gain

Chocolate is one of the worst foods for causing weight gain

Chocolate is:

- High in fat
- High in sugar
- Highly addictive

The combination of these three factors is disastrous for any weight loss program.

Animal fat gives chocolate its smooth texture. Fat is well documented for weight gain.

Sugar supplies the body with empty, low-quality calories and excessive carbohydrates that are converted into body fat. Overeating then becomes necessary in order for the body to obtain enough energy or nutrients.

Addiction of course, makes us want to eat more and more - even if we know we should stop. In other words for people to stay healthy, they have to eat larger amounts of nutrient deficient foods so as to receive the right amount of goodness. This scenario leads to obesity, heart disease, high cholesterol, high blood pressure and ill health. To say nothing of the fact that eating instant sugar leaches high levels of minerals out of our systems, leaving us with more cravings for the food that caused the problem in the first place.

Please note; I am talking about commercial processed chocolate not raw cacao. I do understand that Cacao's in its natural form has good health benefits related to naturally occurring compounds in the bean. Once you have finished Daniel's diet and you want to indulge in making your own healthy cacao treats that is only minimally processed then why not. Cacao is bitter in its natural state so you would add stevia as an herbal sweetener. Recipes using raw cocoa butter and organic coconut oil, cinnamon, vanilla and natural ingredient would be a good way to have sweet treats (after Daniel's diet).

Coffee/Caffeine
To a lot of people coffee is just a beverage to be consumed whenever they feel like it.

Many people say, "I need coffee ...
- To get me started in the morning."
- To give me a lift."

- To calm my nerves."
- To be sociable."
- To stay awake."

But I'm afraid there's more to coffee than just a hot drink.

Coffee is one western dependency drug that seems to get away without the condemnation it deserves. It's already entrenched as part of our culture or social scene, making it acceptable for even young teenagers to meet at trendy cafes to share in this substance.

The essence of coffee addiction - caffeine - is also found in tea, cola drinks, cocoa, chocolate and many pharmaceutical medications. Caffeine is an alkaloid and belongs to a group of methylxanthines, found in many natural plants. Caffeine was a herbal medication until it became commercially sold as a social beverage. The resultant processing creates a class of chemical that, by stimulating the central nervous system, can cause brain and spinal cord disturbances.

After a cup of coffee is finished, the caffeine quickly crosses cell membranes and reaches every cell in the body. The caffeine, in this readily available form, triggers a release of norepinephine – the brains own natural 'feel good' chemical. It makes us feel good and therefore, not only do we want more of it but we also believe it must be good for us. Beware of this common deception. Caffeine, when used appropriately as God made it in nature, is a wonderful herbal stimulant, but not as an excessively used man-made drug.

Two or more cups of coffee per day contain enough caffeine to stimulate the cerebral cortex of the brain, sharpen the senses, distort muscle co-ordination and hamper timing.

Too much caffeine interferes with the normal function of your brain's neurotransmitters. As with sugar and chocolate, caffeine creates an artificial 'high' within the body, which is replaced by a low as the effects wear off. Another cup of coffee eases this feeling but also starts the familiar addiction cycle. Regular interference to your normal brain waves causes the 'need' for more of the artificial stimulant in order to keep feeling normal. This situation creates not only physical health problems but emotional ones too.

Caffeine's addictive properties have been confirmed by many studies and heavy drinkers have been known to experience four distinct signs of addiction:

- Tolerance for the drug/caffeine
- Withdrawal symptoms when it is removed
- A craving or strong desire after deprivation
- Waking up tired, groggy and irritable. Feeling much better after the morning cup of coffee (or tea), because it stops the overnight withdrawal symptoms.

Further symptoms of caffeine overload

- Insomnia
- Energy swings
- Nervousness
- Headaches
- Restlessness
- Constipation or opposite
- Spacing out
- Irritability
- Tremors
- Anxiety
- Cravings
- Raised blood pressure
- Inability to work effectively when deprived
- Heart palpitations and trembling
- Aggravated Irritable Bowel Syndrome
- Spasms in the chest and stomach

Large daily doses of caffeine can affect men and women's fertility and may cause birth defects. During pregnancy high doses of caffeine can cause complications and lower the baby's birth weight.

In my clinic, I regularly treat people who suffer from 'restless legs'. This condition is usually corrected by taking caffeine out of their diet and including Magnesium, Gingko Biloba (an herb) and vitamin E.

How Much Caffeine is in our Beverages and Snacks?

- 1 cup of coffee (8 fl oz) = approx 100-150 mg of caffeine

- 1 cup of tea (8 fl oz)   = approx 40-50 mg
- 1 x 1 oz chocolate   = approx 5-10 mg caffeine
- 1 bottle of caffeinated soda   = 50-60 mg caffeine

250 mg a day is recorded as causing addictive symptoms and is a form of dependency.

This means any more than 1 -2 cups of coffee a day is NOT recommended.

Consultations through my clinic have shown some people regularly consume up to twenty or more cups of coffee a day, six to ten cups a day is very common. I also know that there are many people who drink up to two to four quarts a day of caffeinated soft drinks and 'energy drinks' on top of consuming coffee

A lot of clients tell me they are so used to the caffeine that it doesn't keep them awake at night. This means they have developed a tolerance to the drug. This is a warning sign of addiction. They may suffer from 'caffeinism' – which is a socially accepted form of substance abuse. A non-addicted person may not be able to sleep after drinking only one cup of coffee.

Are you addicted?

Try going completely without caffeine for seven days. After this time, you should be in no doubt, one way or another, as to whether you are addicted. The symptoms will not lie; craving, withdrawals, headaches, irritability, etc, will manifest if you are addicted.

A word of caution here for anyone who consumes large quantities of this drug and wisely decides to give it up - wean yourself off slowly. You don't want to suffer the withdrawal symptoms too severely.

A Cocktail for Disaster: Milk-Sugar-Coffee

Mixing coffee with milk and sugar is a lethal cocktail. After considering what has been said in this section plus what you will read in the milk and sugar section, it should be obvious why! Yet people are regularly mixing three unhealthy ingredients together and drinking it without regard for what is happening inside their body.

This danger doesn't just apply to coffee either, anything that includes caffeine is detrimental, including the cold coffee or chocolate flavored refrigerated milk beverages, which are so popular. They are a Cocktail for Disaster!

Combating the side effects of caffeine:
Drink a large glass of water after each cup of coffee, to prevent dehydration and kidney problems.

Excess caffeine lowers the levels of Tyrosine, a substance vital for production of normal norepinephrine in the brain and for the normal function of the thyroid.

Pre-ground coffee is often rancid by the time you drink it.

Mineral absorption can also be altered; take a multi mineral with Iron (plus C), Magnesium and Calcium.

Please note: People suffering any heart problems, nervous disorders and depression, high blood pressure, irritable bowel, lethargy and osteoporosis should avoid coffee.

Those who are pregnant or planning a baby should avoid all caffeine entirely; as caffeine can have an impact on the growing fetus. It is able to freely pass through the placenta and is transferred through breast milk and one study found that just two cups of coffee ingested during pregnancy may be enough to affect fetal heart development and reduce heart function over the entire lifespan of the child [1]. That is two cups of coffee during the entire pregnancy – not two cups of coffee per day.

'Decaf'
I advise anyone who consumes an excessive amount of coffee to substitute it for a form of coffee that does not have any of the addictive side effects.

By doing this the habitual side of coffee drinking can be broken and eventually the drink replaced with green tea or dandelion coffee. These beverages have, amongst other beneficial health properties, antioxidant properties and low caffeine content. Dandelion beverage, which has more body to it than tea, has no caffeine and is a liver support herb.

Most health food stores carry a range of substitute beverages, which are both satisfying and nutritious, but make sure no lactose or other ingredient is added to them by reading the labels.

This diet is simple really. Substitute anything harmful with something beneficial. By following this process, nobody has to miss out on a social outing or feel left out of social gatherings.

Decaffeinated coffee is ONLY a better choice than coffee if it's naturally decaffeinated. This means decaffeinated by a water extraction method, not by chemical extraction.

The method of extraction should be written on the coffee jar, if not suspect the worst.

I discuss decaffeinated coffee here because of educational purposes – whilst on Daniel's Diet there should be NO Decaf consumption at all. So why not make this a time to change over to dandelion coffee and green tea, both of which are recommended on this diet.

Tea

The average cup of black tea contains:
- 2-5% caffeine, which supplies the stimulating effect
- 7-14% tannin, which gives the color, texture and essential oils for flavor and aroma. The tannins also have some beneficial qualities

Tea should be drunk with a squeeze of lemon and without milk or sugar. In this form, one or two cups a day are not harmful, however during this diet they are not recommended.

Green Tea versus Black Tea

Green tea is the original tea bush in its natural state. It contains powerful antioxidants (mainly Catechins) that are beneficial in the body's fight to combat free radical toxins, cancer [2] and cholesterol. It also helps restore energy, control blood pressure and is beneficial for diabetes. This is proven by the fact that a country where green tea is regularly consumed has a significantly lower percentage of cancer and other illnesses. [3][4].

Black tea is the original green tea bush after it has been cooked or burnt. It also contains the same antioxidants and their properties but, due to the burning process, less of them.

In general terms a good daily intake would be three to four cups of green tea and/or two to three cups of black tea. Ideally all these should be without milk and sugar, but if necessary a small amount of the herbal sweetener Stevia, the natural sugar Xylitol or unprocessed honey can be added.

I personally drink three to four cups of green tea daily, along with other herbal teas. If I am out socially and have no access to green tea, I then drink black tea with a slice of lemon.

It has strong weight loss properties so be encouraged to drink more organic green tea.

Vegetable Oils

Most vegetable oils sold in supermarkets are created by the seeds being chemically treated to extract the oil, requiring that the oil then be heated to an extremely high temperature for the chemicals to evaporate. Unfortunately this intensive heat also destroys much of the nutritional value and according to nutritionists, renders the oil carcinogenic (cancer forming).

However, oils are important to our diet and health and are not manufactured in our bodies so therefore must be included in our diet. This is why they are called Essential Fatty Acids (EFAs). Today the main EFAs are often recognized as Omega 3 & 6 oils.

A lack of them can cause many health problems including:

• PMS   • Skin problems   • Emotional instability

EFAs are beneficial in:

- Lessening blood cholesterol
- Arthritis
- Asthma
- Hyperactivity
- Attention Deficit Disorders
- Inflammatory conditions, like; rheumatoid arthritis, eczema and endometriosis.

The Best Oils for Your Body

Cold pressed oil, contained in dark glass bottles is the best and safest way to buy all oils. Here the liquid has been extracted without the use of chemicals or excess heat. Light and oxygen causes rancidity so that's why storage in dark glass is important. Most oils are preservative-free, but for anyone concerned about the oil going off (rancid), I recommend emptying two capsules of 500 IU of vitamin E oil into the bottle after opening it. Because its powerful antioxidant qualities, will help prevent oxidization and therefore rancidity.

Olive oil has a history of use spanning thousands of years, and the Mediterranean countries that use it regularly experience lower levels of the diseases that are common in America.

Being a monounsaturated fat, and high in oleic acid, olive oil is the most stable oil and therefore a good choice for salads and light cooking. It can also be used as a spread instead of margarine or butter. Very high quality, organic olive oil would be the best choice with the second being extra virgin olive oil. Do not forget Coconut oil, of all the oils it is the most stable (therefore the safest and healthiest) when heated for cooking.

Polyunsaturated fats, which include common vegetable oils such as corn, soy, safflower, sunflower and canola, are **not** to be used in cooking. These omega-6 oils are highly susceptible to heat damage and therefore are not recommended after heating.

Monounsaturated oil like olive oil has some Omega 3 content. Other good sources of monounsaturated oils include almonds and avocado. For this reason, I advise adding half an avocado to your daily foods during this diet, along with almonds.

Flaxseed oil (also called Linseed oil), which contains both Omega 3 - 6 & 9 oils, is a healthy choice and can be used daily on this diet. This oil must be purchased refrigerated and kept in the fridge to ensure its freshness. Alternatively, you can grind your own fresh flaxseed, and this will also have the same benefits. Fish oil supplements are recommended on this diet and can be taken long term, make sure they are not from farmed fish but wild ocean fish.

Margarine – Plastic Fats

Margarine is a man-made food that can contribute significantly to poor health. Nearly all margarines undergo different processes; it's deodorized, artificially colored, flavored and stabilized. It also goes through a process known as hydrogenation. Whilst it makes the oil solid and therefore easier to spread and increases its shelf life, these all creates a so called food that is close to 'plastic' and substances called trans-fatty acids. These act like saturated fats in our body; they stimulate the production of cholesterol

This Trans form of fatty acid is NOT natural. It's a foreign toxic agent and because it has no natural metabolic function, the body doesn't have the capability to handle it. It's also cancer forming and a significant factor in contributing to the creation of gallstones and heart disease [5] [6]. Obviously it is one of the 'bad oils'.

Conclusion

Organic butter is far better (healthier) than traditional margarines. The other problem with margarine is that an artificial coloring agent is added to give it the nice yellow appearance and this additive is not ideal for your long-term health. If you are unsure what you are buying, look on the label it will always give a contents breakdown.

As this diet is a detox program, no butter (animal product) or margarine is permitted but uncooked flaxseed and/or olive oil is a must. Include them individually, or mixed, to your salads and vegetables dishes.

If you react badly (nausea) to raw oils it can be a sign of liver and gall bladder overload, in which case take smaller amounts and use the liver cleansing herbs as an addition to your diet.

Salt

Many people crave salty foods. They must have it in their cooking or added to their meals. Some believe the desire for salt indicates a lack of salt and that their body 'needs' some. This is highly unlikely. It's more likely to be because their taste buds crave the additive taste due to its over use.

The necessary salt or sodium can be found naturally in various vegetables (e.g. celery) to help meet our bodily requirements. Sodium is one of our bodies' necessary minerals or electrolytes. The trouble though, is that table salt is over used causing a possible imbalance in other minerals, leading to health symptoms like water/fluid retention and blocked arteries.

Make sure the salt you buy has no MSG added to it – it's been found added to vegetable salts.

Eating salt is a taste HABIT. Table salt perverts our taste buds into desiring more of it.

Sadly it starts from childhood, from well-intentioned but misinformed parents. This is a lot to do with how we have lost the taste for unadulterated, normal foods.

Our society is in a health crisis. Yet all we have to do to correct this is change back to God's principles for health, which in part are laid out in this book. This diet and educational book can be the key to changing the health statistics in your family and the nation.

Thankfully, taste buds can be re-educated. Simply reduce the salt (and sugar) used in cooking, then lessen the use of the saltshaker. After a few weeks all cravings will pass, leaving taste buds able to once again appreciate good wholesome foods.

Table salt is different to rock or sea salt. Table salt is refined salt. It is a substance, modified by man which like any other chemical additive is absorbed too easily by the body. Table salt is a lot like white sugar; it has found its way into nearly all processed and fast foods.

Natural vegetable, sea or rock salt doesn't go through processing so being more natural substances, are better utilized by our bodies than standard table salt. Coarse ground Celtic salt and Himalayan rock salt is my recommendation – although if it's fine ground it will have less mineral content. Regularly we hear that soils, and therefore all vegetables grown in them, are becoming depleted in trace minerals, so the fact that these salts contain trace minerals should be justification alone for changing to them.

We all need salt or sodium in our diet – it's just a matter of using the right sorts in the right quantities.

Grains

Everyone who wants to lose weight should avoid grains (especially wheat). This is because the grains actually break down to sugar, quickly causing rises in insulin and creating weight gain.

Most people eat bread at least once a day, but more likely two or three times. This combined with the consumption of breakfast cereals, corn bread, muffins, pancakes, cookies, crackers, cakes, pie crusts, pastries, sauces, gravies, pastas and some soups, adds up to excessive amounts of grain and flour in our diet – especially wheat. Over a period of time this continual intake causes health problems.

Much of our land has become an unhealthy growing environment, due in part to modern farming methods, which leaves soil covered with super phosphate, pesticides and herbicides. It doesn't matter in this instance if the grain we eat is whole or refined, eventually digestive overload and food allergies or sensitivities will manifest.

Overcooking and refining of grains destroys the natural enzymes needed for proper digestion and assimilation, causing toxic overload and potential damage to the intestinal area. The result is that larger molecules of undigested wheat particles re-enter the blood stream, causing allergies, overload on the liver and causing multiple health symptoms. Naturopaths call this 'Leaky Gut Syndrome,' or Hyper permeability of the intestinal wall.

Since a lot of the symptoms caused by this scenario appear to have no relationship to bread or other grains they are masked and often recognized as recurring problems.

Consequentially they are also treated as something else. *Some examples of the misdiagnosis are:*

• Intestinal problems	• Brain fatigue
• Depression	• Irritable Bowel Syndrome
• Headaches	• PMS
• Tiredness	• Skin problems
• Constipation	• Irritability

Allergy/sensitivity reactions to grain can often be recognized by strong daily cravings and the need to eat any form of refined carbohydrates, sugars and/or grain products. This urge to eat a favorite food can make it very difficult to stay on diets, especially when our bodies start to crave the food culprit we have just eaten.

Physical symptoms of the allergy can include:

• Stomach pain	• Discomfort
• Gas or bloating	• Insomnia
• Weight gain	• Tiredness

Yet, despite the symptoms, the desire to eat these foods still overrides the warning signs. For example, have you ever eaten a large meal and still wanted something sweet to eat afterwards? You know you can't possibly be hungry but you still 'have' to eat it?

Breakfast cereal, sugar, bread, pasta, pastry and cake are good examples of the foods that cause this   craving or the desire to eat it every day.

Bread

To add further concern, chemicals are used in modern refining and milling methods, and bleaching agents are used to make the bread look nice and white. If you check the food additive code numbers on bread packaging they will show the chemicals added. I come from wheat farming background and let me assure you wheat grain is not naturally white in color, its golden brown.

There is a strong probability that today's bread poses a very real danger to the general population. In the old days dough was made in the evening and baked the next morning, after rising overnight. Now, with quick acting yeast, it can rise in about thirty minutes or even less. It may stay in the oven about the same amount of time, whereupon it's rushed to the cool room where it's soon ready for slicing and packaging.

With such a procedure, you can count on the fact that this bread will be full of live, quick acting yeast, ready to multiply in your alimentary canal.

I still remember vividly, an experiment that I did back in my student days. It was the middle of a typically hot Australian summer (over 100 degrees F) and the whole class was asked to bring in half a loaf of un-sliced white bread. We went outside and, after squeezing the bread in our hands; we laid it down on the hot asphalt. To our surprise it didn't take long for the bread to become a sticky, gooey, white mess.

"This," our teacher exclaimed, "is what sits in your intestines after you eat white bread." "This is the reason for the bloated, constipating lump in your stomach." Interestingly Gluten comes from the Greek word for glue!

Needless to say a lot of the packed lunches brought to class changed after that experiment. In reality what we had bought as white bread was really just heated dough, not baked bread. Here lies the problem. In my opinion everyone should seriously consider giving up white bread, and eat a specially made organic rye bread for example, especially those who suffer from:

- Bloating
- Lethargy
- Intestinal discomfort

- Headaches
- Constipation
- Thrush or 'jock itch'
- Unexplained allergy symptoms

If this wasn't enough, in America today white processed bread is packed full of sugar. We don't naturally consider this, because bread doesn't usually come under the category of 'candy' or 'sweets'.

REMEMBER:

ALWAYS check the labels on the foods you eat – you'll be surprised what seemingly 'harmless' foods actually contain.

In my clinic I see on a daily basis the health benefits of my patients going off grains and bread in particular.

This is why on the Daniel's Diet wheat, cereals and all bread are NO foods.

Case History

A middle-aged man was regularly attending my Daniel's Diet weight loss classes. He had lost 44 pounds (20 kg) and his many health symptoms were dramatically improving. Then, for his birthday, his wife brought him a bread maker.

Within a month he started putting weight back on and his health started reversing back to what it had been before he started the diet. Of course, the man was concerned at the steps backwards in his health, but once we narrowed down the cause to the purchase and subsequent high use of the bread maker, the machine was reluctantly removed from the house and the man's weight and health status improved dramatically.

Dairy Products

I don't eat dairy foods and have, over the years, lost count of how many people I have advised off them.

By so doing, I have seen some near miraculous healings take place, from the disappearance of mucus type problems to increased energy, weight loss to less allergies, clearing of skin problems, constipation fixed, decreased stomach problems and arthritis to name but a few.

It's especially noticeable in children's ailments:

- Unhappiness   • Tummy problems   • Skin complaints
- Ear and nose problems
- Excess vomiting   • Excess crying

Ear infections are often triggered by intolerance to certain foods – milk being the main culprit. The allergic reaction causes swelling and blockages to the Eustachian tubes (the tiny passage connecting ears and throat). This blockage sets the stage for bacterial activity and infections result – enter antibiotics. Antibiotics upset the normal balance of bowel flora causing further complications and upsetting the normal equilibrium in the child.

The addition of a probiotic supplement, Bifidobacteria and Lactobacillus bacteria to the diet are vital at this stage to prevent the imbalance within the body. There are many more varieties of probiotic flora, it is just a matter of finding the right ones to suit your individual needs. Even if it's been years since the original problem I still recommend you take a course of the friendly gut bacteria. Also a multi vitamin/mineral would assist. And don't forget to eliminate cow's milk from the child's diet and the mum's if she's breastfeeding.

Sensitivity symptoms are often camouflaged because dairy foods come under the 'natural food' bracket. As with other foods that we have intolerance to, more often than not the symptoms are masked or blamed on something else.

Do yourself a big favor and limit your dairy intake. [7] [8]

"But Philip, if I go off milk where will I get my calcium from?" This is probably the most frequently asked question I receive, and it's very valid too.

Yes, milk does contain Calcium. Unfortunately, milk is not easy to digest. This is mainly due to the fact that when we leave childhood our ability to make the enzyme lactase, which is needed to digest lactose, diminishes. This is what creates lactose intolerance in a lot of people.

There is another ingredient in milk that causes health problems and that's casein. If you are not one of the 70% of the population who are lactose sensitive then casein may be a problem for you. Symptoms like abdominal pain, cramping, bloating, diarrhea, recurrent colds or infections, mucous chest, bad breath, sinusitis, hay fever, eczema, asthma may all be linked directly or indirectly to dairy foods.

Also I have a theory that once milk has been processed (homogenized and pasteurized) the molecular structure of it is altered (denaturization) to such a degree that our bodies cannot recognize it as a normal food. This leaves us with the debatable question of how much of the calcium in milk can our bodies actually assimilate and utilize.

It takes a lot more than milk and calcium to keep bones strong. We also need substantial amounts of vitamin K (found in dark green vegetables) and vitamin D, Folic acid, Magnesium, Potassium, Boron, Zinc and Phosphorus. Plus a healthy vegetable protein source and weight bearing exercise.

Many people are relying on milk or cheese, red meat or a basic Calcium supplement for their Calcium requirements. This way of thinking can give a false sense of security that may lead to problems in later years. It's worth mentioning here, that excess animal protein (such as that found in milk, cheese and meat) is one contributing factor in osteoarthritis, and this includes low fat or skim milk.

Personally, I find that most osteoporosis sufferers who visit my clinic are, in fact, long-term dairy food and meat eaters. An interesting point and you don't have to have a PhD to work out the mathematics of that equation.

Have you ever wondered why so many suffer from Calcium deficiencies when most people consume some form of dairy product daily? Especially those aged over forty years.

Most patients I see are seriously concerned about their calcium requirements, but very few are worried that they are getting enough exercise to build their bones. Exercise and vitamin D are important in the prevention of postmenopausal bone loss.

Better Food Sources of Calcium

The daily recommended intake for calcium is 800-1200 mg.

By eating wisely, everyone should get enough Calcium from their new diet of fresh fruit, vegetables (all green leafy vegetables contain calcium), salads, nuts and seeds, and especially post Daniel's diet with the inclusion of fish, meat (in moderation), dried figs and free range eggs, which are all high in calcium. The added benefit of obtaining Calcium this way is that all these foods include other vitamins, minerals and flavonoids. All of which are essential to help your body absorb Calcium so that it can build stronger bones. To find out which fruit and vegetables contain Calcium *(refer to the food lists)*

Also natural goat's milk and cheese or sheep's milk is a good choice and worth a try for those with intolerances to cow's milk, post Daniel's diet of course.

Calcium Supplements; are they good or bad for you?

Taking Calcium supplements is a very common practice; however it's wise not to take calcium on its own. Always make sure Magnesium and vitamin D are mixed with it. Calcium and Magnesium help balance each other; they work together inside the body to keep bones strong. Magnesium is the counter balance to excess calcium intake; it will help prevent excess calcium from forming stones in your kidneys and from blocking your arteries. All the minerals need to be in balance of each other, if not different health symptoms will appear. Your bones are not only calcium, but a mixture of minerals. This is why I find hair tissue mineral analysis so helpful in my clinic. From just a tablespoon of your hair the analysis report documents your body's complete mineral status.

Calcium Carbonate is a very common Calcium supplement sold in most pharmacies. Those with low stomach acid (such as post-menopausal women) should avoid this product and use Calcium Citrate instead, because the Carbonates can further deplete stomach acid and they may contribute to kidney stones and increase the tendency towards poor digestion.

Another calcium popular amongst naturopaths is called microcrystalline hydroxyapatite; it is a highly bioavailable calcium [9] and is well absorbed whether taken with or without meals, and is therefore a reliable supplement for long-term use. For those people with recurring kidney stone problems, its better taken with meals. Calcium citrate is more commonly recognized and is also a good form of calcium to take.

I encourage everyone who consults with me to have a hair mineral analysis done so excess or even lack of calcium can be counterbalanced.

Hair Mineral Analysis (HMA):

I regularly analyze hair samples through my clinic (this service is available long distance for anyone in USA, UK, New Zealand, South Africa, Europe, Asia and Australia). Minerals are essential for growth, healing, vitality and wellbeing.

This HMA test enables me to get a complete clinical picture of the mineral status in your body, including toxic minerals.

From this analysis I can clinically advise and prescribe to people anywhere in the world, which is a great way to help people's health and longevity. It is a very simple, safe and non invasive test, taken from a tablespoon of your natural hair. (If you have no head hair then it can be taken from the pubic area). It is a technical clinical analysis; it is NOT a 'new age' test that is often used by new age Naturopaths. Where they take a sample of a few lock of your hair and using a pendulum or perhaps a machine and 'read' your hair and tell you the results.

Every single mineral in the body has an effect on every other mineral in the body. The physical body is made up of minerals which are the basis of all life.

A hair analysis test is an efficient way to obtain a comprehensive and accurate mineral deficiency test.

Hair is the second most metabolically active tissue in the body. The hair represents what is occurring inside the cells of the body. A blood test shows what is happening outside the cell and the waste material being discarded. The hair gives a reading of what is being stored in the body. For example, if mercury is high in the hair, a higher concentration of it would also be found in organs like the kidney and liver.

A **hair analysis** gives a clear picture of a person's health history. **Hair analysis** can indicate vitamin, mineral and nutritional deficiencies as well as heavy metal toxicity. It also gives a picture of your stress levels and metabolism.

All minerals need to be in *balance* for our optimal health; for instance if calcium and magnesium is too low you may have muscle twitches, cramps or trouble sleeping. If sodium and potassium are too high you may have hyperactivity.

A hair analysis is also a powerful guide for parents that are searching for help with ADHD, Attention Deficit or Hyperactivity.

You may request this test from anywhere in the world by simply emailing Philip's clinic at thebridgemanway@gmail.com

What Causes Calcium Depletion In Our Body?

The following are causes of Calcium deficiency:

- hormone imbalance
- alcohol, cigarettes and caffeine
- sodas (due to the excess phosphorus)
- refined sugar (it leaches minerals out of the body)
- excess sodium (salt)
- laxatives, marijuana and general intoxicants
- excess animal protein
- too much, or too little, exercise
- **not enough sunlight (vitamin D)**: Sunshine is God's way for us to internally create Vitamin D, which is imperative for our health. Isn't our Lord so ingenious; we simply stand in the sun light and through our skin Vitamin D is created and delivered to all parts of our body for daily use. The sun is our main source of this essential vitamin and its 'Free. However the biggest word in the Bible is 'if' - if you get enough of the sun.

  Ideally we should all get thirty to forty minutes of sunlight daily, on as much of our skin as possible (40 percent exposure).

Regular sunshine will help our moods and immune system. It's essential for our bone health and helps fight certain cancers (breast, lung, ovarian, colon and prostate). In fact having a vitamin D deficiency may cut your risk of dying in half. [10] Visitors to Australia get so overwhelmed by government and media articles warning of the dangers of Sunshine, so much so that they cover up to the extreme amount and virtually get no sun coverage at all – this is disastrous for your health. Of course getting sun burnt is wrong and unwise and you must use wisdom when in full sun.

Sunlight has great healing potential so don't be afraid of it, just be wise. Also I suggest not wearing sunglasses all the time, only when glare is prevalent because sunlight stimulates the endocrine system as it's filtered through your eyes. I suggest everyone get their Doctor to run a routine Vitamin D test as it is that important. Pregnant women especially should test for D levels as it is imperative for mom and baby's health. In fact everyone should have a blood test done every six months (the test is important because if you are taking vitamin D supplements over a long period of time it is possible to take too much when you might not need it).

When you are tested make sure your reading are high and not low on the test scale. I have lost count of my patients coming to me after they have had a medical test; saying 'the Doctor just said I am ok? When in fact they are not! Your test results show a reference range (51 – 150 nmol/L) in Australia – other countries may differ but the point I am making is the same. Your reading for example may be 60 or even 70 and this tells the Doctor that you don't have a severe deficiency, so they say you are ok. But wait… 60 is still low and there must be a reason it's heading to the minimum of 51. Your health would be far better off it the reading was 140 or closer to the 150 mark. If your reading is up around the 150 mark you don't need supplements – if it's below 100 I suggest you take 4 to 5000 iu's daily and if you suffer cancer or osteoporosis you may have to go to 8000 iu's but seek Doctors advice and have the 6 monthly check up test.

Also check to see what vitamin D you are taking. D 2 (ergocalciferol) is not my recommendation, use only D3 (cholecalciferol), as it is the healthy choice.

Even if you live in a sun drenched country like Australia, but especially if there are long winters in your country or if you cover yourself up excessively from the sun. Please get the test done.

Foods that contain vitamin D 3 are: cod liver oil, soft cooked eggs and fish.

Psalm 139:14 *I praise you because I am fearfully and wonderfully made; your works are wonderful, I know that full well' (NIV).* This is just one small example of the intricate working of our wonderfully made body. But it enhances the need for us to look after our physical body because you and I are wonderfully made; yes *you* are a wonderful person.

Sugar or White Death!

Sugar has been referred to as 'white death', and rightfully so. Eating instant sugars (granulated sugar, processed honey, low percentage fruit juice, cordials, etc) from childhood and increasingly, as we grow older is akin to slowly poisoning ourselves.

Sugar is the main culprit for causing a multitude of health problems, including weight gain and chemical/food cravings.

Many studies have stated that, "Diabetes is epidemic in our society," this is just one manifestation of excess sugar and junk food that is finally being recognized.

The effects from sugar can be subtle and take years to appear.

Therefore they are all too often misdiagnosed and blamed on something else, like:

- Hypochondria
- Emotional problems
- Mental illness
- Weak immune system
- Getting old
- Behavioral problems
- Other illnesses
- Lethargy

Our brain and nervous system require a continuous and regular supply of glucose (natural blood sugar) as much as it needs oxygen. If the flow is insufficient or irregular the brain, energy and nervous system will rise and fall in keeping with the amount of glucose in the blood. Refined carbohydrates and sugar will cause depletion of blood glucose and this is not good for brain energy and function.

If anyone says, refined sugar is natural and therefore good for us, they are misinformed. It's only natural if eaten straight off the sugar cane, sugar beet or direct from the beehive. Raw sugar, taken directly off sugar cane, does have small nutritional value but it was never intended to be processed into a refined additive that is so easily available and over consumed. Molasses is the raw form after its first processing. Sugar granules are the processed form. There is absolutely no nutritional value in refined white sugar, or brown sugar.

It's purely an additive.

Sugar and Weight Gain

Once again, anyone who says sugar is empty calories and therefore not dangerous to a weight problem is missing the facts.

Sugar's quick absorption into our bloodstream causes excess insulin to be released from the pancreas.

On reaching the liver, the excess insulin is converted to triglycerides, which are exactly the form of fats that are stored in all adipose (fat) cells.

To make matters worse, by consuming empty calories your body will demand you eat more and more food to try and supply the lack caused by eating the empty calories in the first place and this is when a vicious cycle of over eating may develop.

Remember raw sugar, brown sugar, processed honey and fruit juices all break down into instant sugars when they are put into your mouth.

Symptoms of Sugar Related Problems
- diabetes, Type 2 (after years of consuming refined sugar, the pancreatic cells often cease to function properly and the first stage of

diabetes can set in). This is very reversible with the right lifestyle and supplements.

- muscle pains, joint pains
- nervousness, irritability, exhaustion
- learning disabilities, hyperactivity (including ADD)
- feelings of weakness when deprived
- lack of sex drive
- faintness, dizziness, tremors, cold sweats
- depression, insomnia and bad nerves
- digestive disturbances and over-acidity (which can cause insomnia)
- orgetfulness, mood swings, anxiety, aggression, violence, anti-social behavior
- phobias, fears
- neuro-dermatitis, skin problems.
- sugar addiction (commonly called a 'sweet tooth')
- mental confusion, limited attention span
- lack of concentration
- itching and crawling sensation under the skin
- eyesight problems, blurred vision, nightmares
- bedwetting in children
- obesity
- poor immunity
- flatulence/gas
- headaches, migraines (often caused by low blood sugar or Hypoglycemia.)
- drunken appearance, as the sugar intake ferments with intestinal yeast it creates a form of alcohol causing unusual brain reactions. This is related to Candida Albicans (yeast fungi, intestinal Thrush or Systemic Yeast Infection.)

The Sugar Story

My children, when they were younger, used to love the story I tell at lectures illustrating what happens inside your body when eating sugar. The abbreviated version is this: I compared every spoonful of sugar we eat to allowing a platoon of enemy soldiers to infiltrate behind our natural defenses. This continual 'guerrilla warfare' deep inside our home territory eventually weakens our army, a.k.a. our immune system and metabolism. Day in, day out, the sugar reinforcements build up. More of the enemy infiltrate with every spoonful we eat. Until, one organ at a time, our body gets overrun. The loss of the battle becomes evident in our own symptoms of ill health.

Quite often, my patients will say, "But I don't eat any sugar!" Yet, when we look closely at their diet, considerable amounts of hidden sugar reveal itself.

Sugar is camouflaged in most packets, tinned and mixed foods. It's labeled under many different names, fructose, lactose, sucrose, dextrose, maltose, and glucose. In fact any ingredient ending with the letters 'ose' is generally a form of sugar. How often have you noticed these not so familiar names listed in the ingredients of 'health' foods? And there we were thinking the food was good for us.

Sugar can be found in most breads, sauces, sodas, fruit juices, health bars, alcohol, and of course most tinned and packet foods. After all, most commercially packaged foods are adulterated with sugars and chemical taste enhancers so that producers can sell more to our growing 'taste perverted' population.

When I was studying for my degree, I remember filling out a class survey on daily sugar consumption. I was very confident of how my results would read. Having made the conscious decision not to add any to my foods, I believed I never ate sugar. Much to my surprise, where I had expected my daily intake to be zero, it was moderate. I had fallen victim to the sugar hidden in so much of our modern foods.

The most common sweetener in your food today!
High-fructose corn syrup (HFCS) is now the most common sweetener used today. Because it comes in liquid form it is easier for food manufac-

turers to use as it dissolves in other liquids, and it is twenty times sweeter than cane sugar, meaning smaller (and therefore cheaper) amounts can be used. Most soft drinks use it and wine, juices, condiments and jello/jams. An average person *eats* about 20 teaspoons of HFCS per day. To make this sugar even worse, the use of mercury-contaminated caustic soda in the production of HFCS is common [11] [12].

Mercury being a very toxic heavy metal is dangerous for everyone, but especially dangerous for pregnant women and small children, whose brains are still developing. I routinely use hair mineral analysis to check for this contaminant and other toxic minerals. So if you are checking food labels remember corn syrup is 'sugar' and put it back on the shelf--especially if it's the first-second or third-highest labeled ingredient

You should be over 18 before being eligible to have a license to eat sugar!

Stress is arguably the greatest health problem in western society today. Excluding addictions from alcohol and drugs, the next greatest problem as I see it is refined sugar. The real tragedy is that our children are eating more and more candy, cakes, sodas and sugary/fatty food.

This is destroying their bodies and minds and setting them up for a life of:
- Diabetes
- ADHD or ADD
- Underachievement
- Tiredness
- Acne
- Headaches
- Poor concentration
- Tooth decay
- Constipation
- Obesity
- Behavioral problems
- Recurring sickness (weakened immune system)

Recently a mother brought her 4 year old child in to consult with me. The child was losing all her front teeth because (her Dentist said), she was given 2 cans of caffeinated soda to drink daily, in addition to other sweets. If this diet and lifestyle is not changed then the future of the child is an unhealthy one. Soda/soft drinks are one of the worst things for you health and weight.

In society today governments have rightfully placed age limits on alcohol and cigarette consumption. However, if the truth were really accepted about sugar, it too would be in this category and have an age limit. This of course will never happen because the topic is politically sensitive, and this view is economically and socially unacceptable - but my point is made. Sugar is a dangerous yet still socially accepted substance.

If we look at past generations, before the modern era, we see that the only sugar eaten was in the form of unrefined carbohydrates like fruit, grains, natural honey and dried fruits with seeds and nuts. In this form the carbohydrates were broken down slowly into simple sugars by the body, which could absorb them at an appropriate rate, avoiding the problems associated with refined sugar.

But even so the book of Proverbs, a book of wisdom has a warning. *"Never eat more honey than you need; too much may make you vomit."* (Proverbs 25: 16 TEV)

Drug like Effect

Refined, instant sugar in all its forms is a powerful chemical agent, for this reason it has a drug-like affect on the body. This is especially true for those people who have developed a dependency on it.

- People who in the morning need: packet breakfast cereals and/or toast and coffee, with 2 sugars.
- People who mid-morning need: cookies, crackers, chocolate, pastry or cake with their coffee (a coffee often taken with cream and sugar
- People who for lunch need: white bread, pasta, soda, white rice

or pastry.

- People who at midafternoon need: more sugar or 'carbs' to overcome hunger cravings (especially chocolate/candy or junk food), lethargy and lapses in concentration.
- People who in the evening need: a sugar or carbohydrate snack, even though they are not really hungry.

Most people consider living and eating like this to be perfectly normal. Sadly, in western society, this is normal, but in the long term it's also extremely damaging, having a negative effect on obesity and both physical and emotional health.

These valueless and harmful foods fill the stomach and provide instant gratification but they often take the place of the real food our bodies need. They fill the stomach and appear to give energy and stimulate the body, but in fact are really just a deceptive decoy; diverting us away from eating the very foods we need for a long healthy life.

Excess sugar and toxins from refined carbohydrates and junk food, inflame, irritate and damage the nervous system, causing erratic thoughts, feelings, behaviour and disorientation of emotional processes. *(Refer to chapter, 'Balancing Your Brain Biochemistry)*

Sugar Makes Us Tired & Dull Minded
When advertisers say sugar is energy they are exploiting a partial truth. Instant sugar is **not energy**, it's only 'potential energy'.

When I hear a parent or sports teacher saying, "Johnny is such an active little boy. I encourage him to snack on sweets and refined carbohydrates because he needs all the energy he can get," I know the adult is misinformed because they are actually harming the child.

Blood sugar (glucose) is very different from refined sugar and sucrose, and it affects the body in quite a different way. Our bodies can manufacture blood glucose from most non-sugar food sources e.g. protein. This natural procedure is done in a regulated, continuous manner depending on the body's daily energy requirements.

Refined sugar on the other hand, by its very nature enters the blood stream like a runaway train (too quickly). This 'rush' of instant sugar floods the bloodstream supplying an instant energy surge, often referred to as a 'sugar boost.' And - yes there is an initial energy increase (the partial truth), but this surge is unnatural and quickly burns itself out. Once the extra supply of insulin has combated the sugar in the blood, it creates a blood sugar drop or a 'downer' (caused by the body's energy level actually being lower now than it was initially). This drop in our blood sugar is the 'hypo' part of hypoglycemia.

It causes:

- Uncontrolled cravings for food - "I need something now! And I don't care what it is'- type feeling.
- 'dullness in the mind'
- loss of energy and tiredness
- ethargy/mood changes
- lack of concentration and memory

The result of routinely eating like this causes people to have sugar intolerance problems.

One of the main ones is called hypoglycemia (low blood sugar) HYPO meaning low, GLYCEMIA meaning sugar in the blood.

Although it's called low blood sugar it's actually brought about by consuming too much sugar and refined carbohydrates. Lots of my patients are told they are hypoglycemic and think that because it's called low blood sugar they must eat more sweets to raise the level again. NO, it's the opposite. Less sweets and more frequent eating of a variety of other good wholesome foods is the answer.

Hypoglycemia and its related health issues are the most common problem I deal with in my clinic. It is at epidemic levels today and causes many health issues.

The sad thing is that a lot of people don't even know they suffer from it and just keep battling on with their lives. As with other food reactions, the symptoms of hypoglycemia become overlooked or masked by other problems and consequently misdiagnosed.

As a result, people take all sorts of medications to fix the symptoms and then more medications to fix the side effects caused by the original medication, and so the cycle goes on.

Those who eat too much sugar travel a roller coaster ride of highs and lows. In my consultations, I have found it's invaluable for patients to understand just what is happening to their body and to recognize the reasons for the symptoms. Most people have little understanding that sugar, caffeine and refined carbohydrates are causing the problem so they continue on totally unaware that they are abusing their own body. I see this as a perception that must be changed, for the sake of everyone's individual future health and well-being.

The danger times:

The main danger times for most people are mid-morning and mid-afternoon –

'The 3-5 PM syndrome': when the cravings, caused by a drop in blood sugar, hit the hardest.

If the need to eat is ignored the results can be quite disastrous:

• Irritability • Over emotional • Starving hungry • Tiredness • Weakness • Impatienc	• Trembling • Loss of concentration • Headaches • Spacing out • Anger

The brain doesn't store energy; it relies on a continual supply from the blood. Your energy is literally 'what you eat'. Lack of nutrient rich, clean, continual fuel means malfunction or no energy. It's as simple as that.

I have suffered hypoglycemia in the past and know most of these symptoms first hand so can spot the signs easily in friends and patients. Let me tell you they are very real, and can mess up your life in many ways.

The key to overcoming it is to eat wholesome natural food, regularly. This will keep your blood sugar at a constant (normal) level, enabling your energy (blood glucose) to come from healthy nutrients in a slow release action, avoiding the chemical ups and downs and side effects. Enabling you to have a focused mind without the need for props. The point is that if your spirit is controlling your flesh as it should be and you are a healthy person, you can choose to indulge occasionally if you want to because you are in control of the choices you make and not dictated to by fleshly desires and addictions.

Sugar Cravings

Stop eating as much sugar, refined carbohydrates and additives as possible. This means sodas, white flour products, white rice, pasta, etc. There are books available that give a list of High/Low Glycemic Index (GI) foods. They simply list all the carbohydrate foods that contribute to rapid rise in blood sugar levels.

Eat at least 5 times a day. This will prevent the blood sugar dropping to a level where cravings for things such as sugar, fast food, caffeine or cigarettes start to manifest. An acceptable snack could be fresh fruit, any salad or raw vegetable juice, seeds, nuts, dried fruit or a cooked meal of vegetables. After the ten days of Daniel's Diet animal protein can be eaten in moderation.

Eat enough dietary fiber. This is very beneficial in the prevention, control and treatment of blood sugar disorders. Fiber slows down the digestion and absorption of carbohydrates, thereby preventing rapid rises in blood sugar. Foods like legumes, brown rice and oat bran, nuts, seeds, most fruits and vegetables, come under this heading as do Psyllium husks.

Regular exercise is also very beneficial in overcoming sugar-related symptoms. You can help decrease body fat by increasing muscle mass with resistance exercise (weights, swimming, physical work etc). One common fact I notice when testing the muscle mass of overweight females is that there muscle mass is nearly always minus.

When they undergo resistant exercise and get their muscles from minus into the plus area then the fat ratios drop dramatically. This can be the key for some women who eat well but find it difficult to lose and maintain weight loss.

Eat protein. It contains amino acids needed by the liver to release stored Glycogen into the blood stream. Eating nuts and seeds and using vegetable proteins in your diet and/or in a shaker supplement can be most helpful.

When I was young I used to have two heaped teaspoons of sugar in my daily six to eight cups tea and coffee. Each day I'd eat half a packet of cookies plus, ice cream or chocolate, white bread, packet cereal with another tablespoon of sugar, and consume alcohol. I changed – so can you.

I enjoy my food much more now than then and if just a pinch of instant sugar was added to my cup of tea, I wouldn't be able to drink it. It tastes revolting.

The advice I give to patients attending my clinic, with regards to cutting sugar from their diet, depends on their individual physical situation, personality and determination.

To those suffering any sort of medical problem I suggest, do it slowly and under supervision. One way is to start by halving your sugar intake for a week or two then halving it again. This process should be repeated until there is no longer any sugar in the diet. For the healthier or stronger personality types I recommend eliminating all sugar immediately.

There is no doubt that anyone cutting addictive foods from their diet will experience cravings. It will be tempting to stop the withdrawal symptoms by eating the desired or culprit food. After all, it will stop the cravings, and whilst this might seem to imply that the food is actually good to eat, in the long term as we are now learning, the opposite is true.

If you are determined in your mind to change and fight through the cravings, it won't be long before they ease. Then your taste buds will revert back and you will start seeing and feeling the positive results of the diet, and what's more you'll enjoy all the natural tastes and flavors from your food.

If the cravings are strong it may take some determination to overcome them but it's well worth the effort. The supplements below will definitely assist in all dietary changes and let's face it, any help is worthy of consideration. I strongly recommended the use of these supplements.

Warning on 'Diet' Products!

The most common of theses 'diet products' are diet sodas, snacks, sweets, table top sweeteners, chewing gum and diet yoghurts. They contain artificial Sweeteners including Splenda (Sucralose) and Aspartame (NutraSweet) and Saccharin.

They may seem a good alternative to their high calorie counterparts, but don't be misled, they are unhealthier in the long term. Why? Because they are laced with 'artificial' or chemical sweeteners and create a toxic reaction inside us - DO NOT consume them on Daniel's Diet. As the name 'artificial' suggests, they are completely unnatural. It is possible to actually increase weight gain when using chemical sweeteners.

People who are addicted to sweet things and consequently sick from this lifestyle of eating too much sugar and refined carbohydrates in the first place need to get away from the dangerous sweet foods and eat more 'real' foods – the natural foods God created in the first place.

An important part of Daniel's Diet's success is to break people away from wanting to gratify the sweet cravings and to change their taste buds to wanting good wholesome foods. By eating artificial sweeteners we are encouraging people to still desire the wrong foods. They actually increase your craving or desire for refined carbohydrates.

By promoting these artificial sweetened foods as 'diet foods' we are giving a 'False Sense of Security' and by eating them you are not going to become healthier because the cause of the problem is not only being ignored but encouraged. In fact these sweeteners could be more harmful and addictive than sugar itself [13].

Artificial sweeteners are 'sold' to us as the sugar substitute which has low calories and therefore ideal for weight loss. However research is revealing that they upset the body's natural satiety response and increase hunger. Artificial sweeteners therefore can cause weight gain overall [14]. An abject lesson for me recently was when a long term patient of mine whom I had successfully treated for Chronic Fatigue Syndrome (CFS) rang me with this story.

He recently went on vacation so he decided to relax and eat and drink things that he had given up over the duration of his treatment for CFS and depression. He drank 2 bottles of 'diet soda' a day and 1 cup of coffee with cake. His self talk was, ' I am feeling better now and while on vacation – why not indulge a little - this was not too excessive'. However after 3 days the old symptoms of CFS started to manifest. He felt so tired and lethargic that he had to lie down and sleep several times a day and all night. Anxiety rose up in him and a depressed heaviness filled his mind. It was a 'weird, spacey' feeling he explained. After 2 more days he stopped drinking the soda (and coffee) and within 24 hours all those symptoms left him. His words were 'it just had to have been the chemicals in the diet soda.'

The problem in diagnosing chemical reactions like this is that most times the presenting symptoms are initially ignored or blamed on something else.

Supplements to Help
Chromium

Chromium is a trace element, required for the successful metabolism of sugar. With it the body can manufacture the 'glucose tolerance factor' or GTF, which regulates the blood sugar. Since sugar robs our bodies of Chromium, this mineral is a necessary supplement. It's of special importance to diabetics, sugar cravers (those with a 'sweet tooth') and those who are hypoglycemic but also to those who crave savory food.

Zinc

Zinc is a constituent of insulin and is required by the body for many things, including the healing of all tissues. It's grossly deficient in the western diet, and is essential for hypo and hyper – Glycaemia.

Gymnema Sylvestre

Gymnema Sylvestre, literally meaning 'sugar destroyer' is an excellent herb for reducing appetites and sweet cravings. Gymnema extract is very beneficial for the control of obesity.

For this reason, it's highly beneficial to diabetics and those with hypoglycemia. If you have a 'sweet tooth' - this is the herb for you, in combination with the trace mineral Chromium.

Scientific research has found that it also reduces the appetite for up to ninety minutes after its sweet-numbing effect.

How Gymnema works as an appetite suppressant is not known. One thought is that its effect on the taste buds creates a nervous reflex that modifies the appetite centre in the brain. This effect is subtle, and will work best with consistent use.

Healthy Sugar Substitutes

Stevia is an herb and a safe form of sweetener. It's better than any artificial sweetener used in diet foods and drinks, and it can be used in moderation by hypoglycemic. It does have a slight 'metallic taste'. Diabetics should check with their doctor first but it should be safe for you too.

Unprocessed honey in moderation may be used, but keep in mind it is high GI (sugar). However I am encouraging you to try and go without all sugar at least on this 10 day diet plan.

I would like to reiterate here that, in order to succeed, you must want to change and give up some foods, even if you love eating them. Your mind and emotions play a big part in finding the strength to overcome the cravings. I sometimes hear people complain, "the herbs don't seem to be helping." It's obvious in these situations that, at a deeper level, there is a much bigger issue than food addiction, which needs addressing. The herbs are not miracle workers (only Jesus does that), but they are very helpful and necessary to assist in the journey towards better health.

Yet, even once the cravings are beaten, there is often another problem; a strongly ingrained habit that goes with sugar addiction. I used to eat sweets and candy whenever I watched TV or when I was bored or lonely and, whilst after time I actually lost the desire for candy, my mind still looked for them out of habit.

However, with the help of the minerals, herbs and then the positive results of feeling much healthier, more energetic, motivated and losing weight, you will realize that it's worth it. Sometimes we just have to be tough and say "NO".

Danger Foods for Sweet Tooth's!
- most commercial breads
- most packet cereals
- white flour products, like cookies and crackers (sweet and savory), cup cakes, muffins, donuts
- white rice
- refined sugar and refined carbohydrates
- pastry
- processed pasta
- sodas and fruit juice concentrates

The above foods are the Number One enemies in our fight for good health and weight loss.

Keep in mind that these foods are refined carbohydrates and once eaten break down into instant sugar within your system. So they are no different to straight up candy.

Would you eat Pudding for breakfast and pretend it was healthy?
When you or your children sit down to breakfast with a bowl of packet cereal, it is no different to you eating a bowl of sweet pudding. I know some people may question this. We have been told through advertising that breakfast cereal is a good way to start the day. Yes, whole grains

are good for you (these are called complex carbohydrates) and eating a proper breakfast is very important. However, the high sugar loading of most commercial cereals is not good for you and outweighs any use. What happens is when the cereal reaches your stomach it breaks down into sugar, just like if you ate a piece of cream cake.

Some whole grain cereals are sugar free; make sure these are your first choice, when having cereal. (This advice is for after Daniel's Diet as there are to be no breakfast cereals at all on this diet).

Please note: This information is a guide only. Each individual will have different foods and situations, but the principle remains the same

CHAPTER TEN

IS DANIEL'S DIET NUTRITIONALLY BALANCED?

We only have to look at the diet's original source to find the answer is YES!

"Well at the end of the 10 days, Daniel and his three friends looked healthier and better nourished than the youths who had been eating the food supplied by the king."
Daniel 1:15 (TLB)

Alternatively this could read,

"Well at the end of the 10 days... (enter/say your name) looked and felt healthier than all the other people around them who were eating the junk food freely available in modern society."

The 10-day program is especially formulated to cleanse your system and, where appropriate, help you lose weight safely. Most diets that encourage quick weight loss are not recommended because they are concerned with only weight loss and not health. That is why this 10-day program is so powerful and unique, because it's a detox program - designed to help bring the body back into balance. Weight loss is merely a wonderful side effect.

The Power of Food

Food is a weapon - it can be used for you or against you.

Natural foods have been created to be the only true source of our energy supply. Indeed they are our life's supply line. They have the exact ingredients we need for an abundant healthy life, from the cellular level outwards. There's more than enough evidence showing that eating more vegetables and fruit is the single most important dietary change needed to reduce disease.

On the other hand, man adulterated (processed) food contains ingredients that are a weapon towards our own destruction.

The specific properties found only in fruit, vegetables and seeds are so powerful that they fight, and often win, the war against cancer and most disease. There have been countless reported incidents to prove this; Cases where people suffering from different illnesses and diseases have returned to good health, simply by adapting their lifestyle and diet to include natural foods, mainly from the plant kingdom.

Case History

Jim, (a cancer patient) had been medically diagnosed and treated for this disease. His family brought him to me because they were desperate. The prognosis was grim. He was emaciated, weak and in constant pain. He had recently finished chemotherapy.

I put him on Daniel's Diet with a supportive herbal regime and a specific rebuilding protein and vitamin supplement.

Two months later, Jim was back playing nine holes of golf.

Four months later, he said, "I feel better now than I did thirty years ago."

One year later, he showed me the golf trophy he had won (over eighteen holes by this time). He was bubbling over with enthusiasm for his pain-free life and newfound lifestyle.

Naturopaths don't treat the disease.

They simply offer the necessary ingredients to enable the body to repair itself and fight off illness.

God has designed our bodies to heal themselves 'if' we just use the potential he supplied us with. Our bodies regenerate continually. Every thirty days for example, our skin is completely renewed.

In other words, if we closely follow the principles of Gods health plan, our body can go from being in a diseased state to being a rejuvenated healthy body in only twelve months.

Food from God's Garden
Fruits, vegetables, seeds & nuts

These are all foods from God's garden. They are the foods that give us unlimited health and life. They contain all the ingredients and nutrients we need for our very existence. These are the foods that should make up 75–80% of our daily diet.

They contain (to name just a few):

- Antioxidants, which help neutralize and eliminate oxidants (toxins) from our bodies.
- Carotenoids, a group of yellow, orange and red substances found in a wide variety of foods. One of these is beta-carotene, which is excellent at stimulating the immune system to fight off viruses and infections.
- Phytonutrients, unique chemicals essential for optimal health and disease prevention
- Lycopene, found in tomatoes and bright red fruits and vegetables, is a nutrient with positive effects on prostate health and significantly reduces the risk of cancer.
- Bioflavonoids, the complex natural nutrient that gives food their colors and flavors. They are important for treating and preventing common health problems.
- All the vitamins and minerals needed for maximum health.
- All necessary amino acid (protein) which when eaten in the right combinations and quantities. No one vegetable contains all the amino acids, so variety is necessary.
- A very high water content, which means they are constantly nourishing and cleansing our bodies.
- All the essential fatty acids can be found in foods like: flaxseed, evening primrose oil, blackcurrant juice, green leafy vegetables, avocado, nuts and soybeans.
- No (or very little) saturated fats or cholesterol making it hard for diseases to multiply.

ALSO...

Their high water content and low fat levels make them perfect for weight loss. Only raw fruits and vegetables contain those vital enzymes, needed to assist in food digestion and the very life of our cells.

Most fruit and vegetables have the necessary enzymes built into them to be able to digest themselves, especially pineapple and papaya. Both of these fruits contain specific enzymes that aid our general digestion, so I recommend that these should be eaten regularly

An example of the Power of food and why we should eat more food from God's Garden: I rate Curcumin, also known as turmeric as one of the top (if not the top) herb or spice for health and as a weapon against disease. It's far more than just a taste enhancer, so please use it as much as you can in your cooking.

Turmeric: whose active ingredient, curcumin, is beneficial for both brain health and cancer prevention or treatment? It has potent antioxidant and anti-inflammatory properties. Another bioactive compound in turmeric is aromatic-turmerone which also has wonderful health benefits. One study shows that curcumin and isoflavones inhibit breast cancer cell growth by 95%.[1]. Another example of its power is indicated in this study on Curcumin and Isoflavones; they inhibit Breast Cancer Cell Growth by 95% [2])

Are all fruit and vegetables healthy?

I must clarify a few points about fruit and vegetables. In an ideal world, as it was back at the time of creation, all foods were organic and fresh and they supplied all the necessary nutrition, end of story.

However, the twenty-first century is not so ideal. And the question often asked is, "Do we really get all the nutrition we needs from natural foods?"

The answer is technically yes, BUT with the ideal fast disappearing, it's not as straightforward as it should be. To gain all the necessary nutrition, we must obtain more knowledge on what foods to eat and what foods not to eat. This is the information that will improve and lengthen our lives. Now is not the time to bury our heads in the sand.

My aim in this book is to educate people, because information and application will empower them to success. Any change, even 30 or 40% is still going to be of great benefit to the individual's health and weight control.

It is possible to rely on your diet for its source of nutrients, but you have to work at it and use 'wisdom for health'.

Biodynamic and Organic Foods
Biodynamic and organic farming are part of the solution needed to avoid nutrient deficiencies and toxins accumulating in our bodies. Biodynamic means the food is grown in soil that has been specially and naturally prepared over many years. Producers have certified proof of this fact. It means toxic chemicals have never been used in the current growing process or in recent years on the soil.

Biodynamic is the most natural and chemical-free way to grow food. It's as close to eating in the Garden of Eden as we can get; the kind of food that, according to the Bible, sustained humans in a time when they normally lived several hundred years. The soils are not only toxic chemical free but have all the minerals in them that are essential for health and longevity of life. Produce grown in them will taste much better because of the nutrient rich soil, nothing like the anemic fruits and vegetables like we get in our stores today.

Organic on the other hand, means that no chemicals have been used whilst growing the current plants. The soils however, may have been sprayed with chemicals more than once during previous years. This is the second best, and most available, healthy food choice. These types of natural foods supply the majority of nutrients that we need. In the United States there has been an 80% increase in consumption of organic food in the last decade, one policy I hope Australians will follow. Organic Fruit and Vegetables are higher in phytochemicals [3] (the good plant nutrients) than general fruits and vegetables. To be sure of what each food contains and how it is produced, food labels need to be read carefully and questions need to be asked.

Fresh, frozen, tinned – which is best?
Obviously fresh is best. Frozen is often more convenient and permissible. Tinned is not permitted on this 10-day program and is, in general the third choice, mainly because of the additives it contains.

Genetically Engineered (GE) or Genetically Modified (GM) Foods
Avoid all food that is Genetically Engineered.
This is food produced using technology and science. GE is a process used to transform a wholesome, natural food into a product, which is more consumable and therefore more financially viable for manufacturers (money before what is best).

This is the general marketing ploy to fool society into believing it's good for us. In most cases, the food's *"re-creation"* involves combining genes from different plants, animals or microbes until the desired result and sale ability is achieved.

For example, to slow the ripening of tomatoes, and to give them a longer shelf life, fish genes have been added to a Genetically Engineered hybrid and to enable certain forms of soybeans to become immune to mass sprayed chemical herbicides, their genes are combined with a bacterium, a virus and a petunia plant.

It's like a plot for a new 'Frankenstein' movie. There are grave concerns at this moment in Australia about the contamination of ordinary canola oil crops by counterpart GE grown canola oil crops.

There are two sides in this GE debate - the multinational companies against the consumers (us). I suggest you think very carefully about which side you take because any decisions in favor of GE, GMO or GM (all meaning the same thing) have the potential to be catastrophic for future generations. Remember the tobacco industry claimed that tobacco doesn't harm health. Scientists certified these claims despite knowing the truth. When big profits are to be made, ethics and morals are ignored. Other examples are asbestos, DDT, and thalidomide. Genetically modified organisms (GMO) will be much worse because it's in our food chain and so eventually you will not have a choice and won't even know in most cases if you are eating this insidious food. The consumer, with their individual spending power, is the only one who can stop this nightmare from unfolding.

On this matter, the Bible quite clearly says, *"And the earth brought forth grass, the herb that yields seed according to its kind, and the tree that yields fruit, whose seed is in itself according to its kind. And God saw that it was good."* (Genesis 1:12)

From this I understand that food was created perfectly, accordingly to its own kind. This surely was not done so that man could change it into a food 'not' according to its own kind. If God thought that his creation was 'good' who are we to change it?

"And look! I have given you the seed-bearing plants throughout the earth, and all the fruit trees for your food." (Genesis 1:29 TLB)

The Power of Fruit

ALL varieties of seasonal fruit should be eaten, especially those grown locally. They supply multiple minerals, vitamins, enzymes, natural sugar and fiber. Eat whatever fruit is in season in your location.

Fruit juices are not acceptable on this diet, as they contain too much concentrated sugar. Orange juice can also cause an adverse sensitivity reaction in a lot of people.

Lemons, however, are different; whilst they are naturally acidic, when they enter the stomach they actually help the body to alkalize and stimulate proper digestive function.

What Nutrients Are Found In Your Fruits?

- **Apple:** an apple a day really may keep the doctor away. Calcium, Iron, Bioflavonoids, some vitamin B's, Boron, polyphenols, Magnesium, Silica, Pectins (found just under the skin). Always eat the skin to get the full benefit and even the seeds are nutritious.

- **Apricots:** Contain antioxidants, Beta Carotene, Folate, Iron, vitamin C, Potassium
- **Avocado:** Is a very low sugar fruit, a single-seeded berry native to Mexico it is one of my favorite fruits. With its proven ability to quell hunger pangs because of its healthy monounsaturated fat content, the avocado is arguably a perfect dietary staple for weight loss. Also contains Essential Fatty Acids (EFAs), Calcium, Iron, vitamin B6, C & E, Magnesium, Zinc, Copper, Folic acid and more Potassium than banana.
- **Bananas:** This lovely tasting fruit does have high sugar content so if wanting to lose weight keep this in mind. It has great nutrition factors of Potassium, vitamin A, B6 & C, Calcium, Magnesium, Phosphorus
- **Cherries:** They are rich in anthocyanins, compounds linked to reduced inflammation associated with heart disease and arthritis and gout. I often prescribe Pure Cherrie juice to gout and arthritis patients. They also contain a powerful antioxidant, which help reduce free radicals in the body, possibly reducing the risk of some cancers. Plus Calcium, vitamin C, Bioflavonoids, Iron, Copper, Manganese
- **Watermelon:** Watermelon is one of the most popular summer fruits because of its cool tasty liquid flesh. Watermelon has a high water content and this is good because eating watermelon on a hot summer day is a tasty way to help you stay hydrated. This fruit in particular is best eaten on its own and never mixed with any other foods as it overloads the tummy when mixed. Many people underestimate this fruit because of its high water content.

However it is one of the most nutritious of them all. Just some ingredients Lycopene, L-arginine, C, A, B6 and magnesium and minerals. I encourage you to eat the seed and rind as they contain many nutrients as well, like iron, zinc, fibre and protein. I am much opposed to genetically modified foods so I am glad to say that seed less watermelons are not the result of genetic engineering. Seedless watermelons are the result of hybridization [4]

- **Dates:** Undoubtedly a favorite sweet fruit since the Garden of Eden. Contains; Iron, Potassium, vitamin K, Calcium, Selenium, magnesium and some B vitamins.

- **Figs:** Another popular and nutritious fruit mentioned in the Bible. Figs are high in fiber like all fruits and contain essential minerals, including magnesium, manganese, calcium, copper, and potassium as well as vitamins, K and B6.

- **Grape Fruit:** Great for weight loss diets in also has Calcium, vitamin C and A, Potassium, Magnesium, Pectins, Biotin. Note: eating grapefruit may, in rare cases, interfere with certain medications, so you may want to discuss this with your doctor.

- **Kiwifruit:** This one is for my New Zealand friends, where it got its name from in honor of New Zealand's native bird. It was introduced by missionaries into New Zealand in the early 20th century from china. It has very high levels of vitamin C and K. It has vitamin A, B6, E, and Potassium.

- **Papaya:** Naturopathicaly speaking I love Papaya or 'paw paw' for its low sugar content and digestive enzyme known as papain along with fibre which helps improve your digestive health. Juicing this truly wonderful fruit is one of the pleasures of eating health. Plus, Calcium, vitamin C, Potassium, Arginine, Beta Carotene and Iron.

- **Peaches**: Contain many nutrients including antioxidants; Beta Carotene (vitamin A), plus multiple minerals and vitamins

- **Pears:** Contain very high fibre content and is a moderate low Glycemic Index fruit which is helpful on a weight loss diet.

- **Pineapple:** are well known in naturopathic circles for their Digestive enzymes; Bromelain, Iron, Potassium, Manganese, Calcium, Iodine, Magnesium, folic acid, vitamin A, B's & high in C

- **Blueberries and Strawberries:** Have low Sugar content and contain flavonoids in the berries known as anthocyanins, which are antioxidants that give these fruits their characteristic red and purple colour. Also Potassium, vitamin C, Bioflavonoids, Calcium, Silica

- **Tomatoes:** Lycopene - (great for helping fight prostate cancer), vitamin C, Potassium, vitamin A.
- **Coconut:** I will sum this fruit up by simply saying it is one of the most nutritious foods of all. Drink the coconut water for its wonderful electrolyte content and is way better/healthier than the sports drinks available.

Eat the Seeds

Have you ever wondered why sweet grapes have bitter seeds?

Most people choose not to eat the seeds found in fruit such as grapes, apples and watermelons. When was the last time you ate pomegranates which have the bitter sweet flavour. I actually asked this question at a seminar and out of the 250 people only one had eaten this fruit in the last year and some younger people had never heard of it. Pomegranate is a very Biblical fruit and has Anti- Cancer Properties. [5]

However, there is a key issue to learn in this combination of sweet and bitter.

Both flavors have valuable nutrients to offer the body. Today we eliminate most bitter parts of the food chain, yet, they contain strong healing agents. Bitter apples, onions, Brussels sprouts, radishes, lemons, etc. all have their individual nutrients that cause the bitter taste. You can buy supplements of grape seed extracts and pomegranate juice from health stores, for medicinal purposes. The point is that if we eliminate bitter foods from our diet we are missing out on the counter balance it brings to fighting off disease.

What Is In Your Nuts, Seeds & Dried Fruit?
Lots of wonderful nutrients:

- Almonds - Vitamin A, B's & C, Calcium, Phosphorous, Magnesium, Iron, Zinc
- Bitter Fruit Seeds -Vitamin B17

- Brazil Nuts - Calcium, Vitamin E, EFA's, Phosphorus, Selenium
- Buckwheat - Calcium, Magnesium, Iron, Bioflavonoid, Potassium and Zinc
- Cashews - Magnesium, Iron, Vitamin E, Calcium, EFAs
- Flax Seeds - EFA's (essential fatty acids), Vitamin E and Silica
- Hazelnuts - Calcium, Vitamin E, EFA's, Iron, Potassium, Selenium and Zinc
- Pecans - Calcium, Vitamin E, EFA's, Magnesium, Potassium, Selenium, Zinc
- Pine Nuts - Iron, EFA's, and Vitamin E
- Pistachio Nuts - Lutein, Beta-carotene Iron, EFA's, Vitamin E
- Pumpkin Seeds - Zinc, EFA's, Calcium, Iron, Vitamin A & B's
- Rice (Whole Grain) - Vitamin B's, Selenium, Magnesium, Calcium
- Sesame Seeds - Calcium, EFA's, Vitamin E
- Sunflower Seeds - Zinc, Calcium, EFA's, Vitamin E, Selenium
  (Essential Fatty Acids is abbreviated to EFA's)

All fruits and seeds are recommended because they are packed with vitamins, minerals and Essential Fatty Acids (EFA's). Most have antioxidant qualities too. I want to single out just a few to encourage you to eat more of them whilst on this diet and in the long-term - especially almonds, pumpkin seeds and sunflower seeds.

- Almonds are of great value in our food chain. Try soaking them in water overnight, before eating them, it aids digestion. Lightly roasting them makes a good treat. One cup of almonds contain approximately 26 g of protein, as well as Oleic Acid, Copper, Calcium, Magnesium, Zinc, vitamin E, EFA's, Iron, Potassium, Selenium and Arginine.
- Pumpkin Seeds are high in minerals especially Zinc and Calcium and every male should eat them daily to aid their reproductive system and prostate.

Case Study

One male patient I advised to eat a handful of pumpkin seeds every day swears that they are a major part of the reason he is a very virile and active sixty-three year old. His hair is actually white but with the inclusion of colloidal minerals to his diet, it's noticeably changing to the original black color.

Vegetables Have It All

Vegetables contain all the necessary nutrients needed for us to function at our peak ability. They contain all the vitamins, minerals, proteins, carbohydrates, essential fatty acids, antioxidants, fiber and enzymes to supply and balance our body's daily nutritional needs. They even contain phytonutrients that balance our hormones and other substances that today's scientists are only now discovering as beneficial. **To receive all the benefits it's vital that we eat a wide variety of vegetables every day.**

Variety is the spice of life, someone once said and it's certainly true in the sense of our eating. Food is to be enjoyed and experimented with. If you walk into a well-stocked vegetable shop, there will be many different fruit and vegetables on show. Chances are that many of them you may know by name but have never tasted. Next time, why not buy one you have never, or only rarely, tasted.

The Colors of the Rainbow

Every colour in every food type from 'God's garden' have individual or unique biochemical health benefits—that is why I always encourage rainbow salads in all my programs and do include recipes for them.

All varieties of vegetables are allowed on this diet whether they are in their natural form or in juices. Whilst bearing in mind the wisdom of not overeating, there is no limit to how many you can eat. It's worth remembering also that every different color vegetable has different nutrients to offer. This is why variety is vital.

In fact, the very chemicals that make foods good for us are the ones that give them color, turning spinach green, blueberries blue and mangoes orange. Therefore make your salads the colors of the rainbow and you will be eating a more balanced diet.

Some examples:
- Yellow & orange - Beta Carotene, Carotenoids
- Red - Lycopene, Beta Carotene, Bioflavonoids, vitamin A & C
- Blue- contain compounds called anthocyanins, phytochemicals that belong to the flavonoid family helping fight off cancer and aid your brain function.
- Green - Chlorophyll and Iron, Calcium, Cobalt, Folic Acid, Iron, vitamin A, B6, & K, Beta Carotene Manganese, Magnesium, Molybdenum, Potassium, Para Amino Benzoic Acid (PABA). Spinach, kale and collard greens have these nutrients plus phytochemicals, lutein and zeaxanthin which ward off macular (eye) degeneration.

The Cruciferous Family

Cabbage, Brussels sprouts, broccoli and cauliflower all deserve a special mention and should be added into your daily diet. They contain natural phytonutrients (phytochemicals), Indoles, enzymes, antioxidants, and numerous vitamins and minerals. They also aid hormone metabolism and can help fight off cancer.

Beans/Legumes

All legumes (the bean family, lentils, red clover, chickpeas) are recommended. So why not enjoy the variety? Legumes are full of isoflavones, vitamins and minerals, which are beneficial in creating normal hormonal balance in men and women. Soaking beans and legumes before cooking aids in their digestion and neutralizes the mineral-binding phytic acid they contain.

Soya beans are a source of protein; they also contain minerals like Calcium and Amino acids.

Soya milk however is not allowed during this diet. Despite it being a natural food and containing good nutrients there is a lot of debate regarding its affects on certain health issues.(I discuss this in detail in my second book).

Avocado is an alkaline food, high in Amino acids. It contains very little sugar and is good for anyone suffering stomach problems. It's full of minerals and some vitamins, is very nutritious, blends well with different menu combinations and is easily digested.

A lot of people avoid avocados because of the belief that they are high in fat. But the fat is easily assimilated and the oil is not a saturated fat but a good oil (part of the essential fatty acids) which the body will utilize, not convert into extra fat cells.

Beetroot (Beets)

The wonderful dark purple color of this vegetable contains numerous ingredients that help detoxify blood and support the liver. It replenishes vitamins, minerals, natural enzymes and natural sugars. For this diet beets should be bought fresh, not tinned or bottled, and eaten either raw or steamed.

It is suggested that anyone with cancer, or anyone wishing to prevent cancer, should consume beets daily. It contains compounds that fight against the disease and inhibits tumors.

Half a juiced beetroot, mixed with carrot juice is a good natural supplement. Alternatively, for those who haven't a juicer, or the time to juice, Beetroot crystals (powder) or tablets can be bought as a supplement.

If there should be any feelings of nausea after having this (or any) juice, it's probably because the drink is too strong for your stomach. In which case water it down and drink smaller doses over the day. Remembering as with any treatment, if any abnormal side effects appear, stop the treatment and find out why. You can test it yourself with wisdom or consult a practitioner.

Carrots, these are a powerful antioxidant and are one of nature's best sources of natural Beta carotene, which when assimilated into our bodies' converts into vitamin A. Carrots also increase energy, stimulate healthy bones, eyes, skin, hair, circulation, colon care, mucous membrane and can be a natural solvent for ulcerous and cancerous conditions. They also contain Phytoalexin, which is beneficial for any one suffering with a yeast infection (Candida Albicans) or thrush.

Please note: Carrot contains the alkaloid Daucarine, which whilst being good for our bodies can, after consistently high doses, add a yellow tinge to the skin. This reaction shows a possible overload of the alkaloid on the body. If this happens it's advisable to lower your intake of Daucarine by eating fewer carrots and stopping any vitamin A supplements. After these changes have been made it should only take a few days for the yellow tinge to disappear.

The Power of Vegetable Juices

I know that not everyone has access to a Juice Extractor so this section is optional. However, I most strongly recommend juicing, as it is a powerful step towards the goal of good health.

In modern day natural therapies raw vegetable juices have always been used and recommended as part of body cleansing and detox programs. They are used to aid our healing system in its fight against many ailments and chronic complaints.

Juicing is powerful because:

It creates a concentrated drink of readily available nutrients, antioxidants and enzymes, which in turn provide an excellent and effective method for cleansing.

By removing the pulp from vegetables we allow our bodies to quickly assimilate the nutrients into our systems. This avoids digestive problems and provides the fastest way to nourish our cells, create energy and rebuild the immune system and bodily organs.

Vegetable juices contain instant energy and detoxification principles; drink two glasses per day.

Always wash the vegetables thoroughly before juicing. Remove any moulds or damaged parts (your body deserves the best) .You can use vinegar in the water to help cleanse or peel the produce if need be. Ofcourse using organic vegetables helps stop any surface toxic chemical concerns.

Which Juicing Machine is best?

All Juicing machines are beneficial; however like most machines there are levels of efficiency. When choosing a "Juicer" the more modern ones are best. They operate at a lower speed, are quieter, squeezing and pressing the fruit or vegetable. Often called "Press Juicing" the slow squeezing (pressing) action of this juicer separates the juice from the pulp without damaging the living enzymes. If you are used to a traditional juicer which spins very fast and liquefies the vegetable and then change to a Press type Juicer you will notice that it goes slow and actually grinds or pulverizes the produce into a more dense liquid. All juicing is beneficial and by adding them routinely into your lifestyle you are well on the way to a healthy body and mind.

SPECIFIC JUICE RECIPES FOR HEALING SUPPORT

In my clinic I recommend specific juices to aid healing. They may be had daily and with any diet plan. Here are just three examples: For more recipes (especially my ' Philips Green Smoothie') see my book 'Daniel's Way Recipe Guide'. Or you can upload the eBook from my web site.

1. Detox (my personal recommendation on Daniel's Diet)
Ingredients
1-2 carrots – depending on size
½ raw beetroot (red beets)
1 celery sticks (stems)
1 tablespoon of blue berries (frozen)
1 stem of spinach
Ginger to taste
½ lemons squeezed
Also if possible add Chlorella (organic). Start with 1/3 tsp and increase if you wish to 1 tsp after you get used to the powerful taste of this smoothie. Chlorella is a natural green algae and an amazing food; it is

chlorophyll rich, has high nutrient value. It is easily digested and high in protein, amino acids, beta carotene and B vitamins.

Chlorella is excellent for detoxing and I use it regularly in my clinic with hair tissue analysis. It has a unique ability to bind to heavy metals and various toxins in your body, and then when it binds to the toxin it has the amazing power to extract these toxins that have been building up in your bloodstream and tissue and helps you eliminate and detox your body.

Other benefits of this juice:
• helps your digestive and bowel health
• Helps bad breathe (and other body odours)
• Helps lower Cholesterol
• Helps Acne and unhealthy skin appearance
• Helps Energy

Note: your stool (bowel movement) may turn red or dark green due to beetroot (red beet) colour or greens. This is normal and not a health problem and will go away if you stop the juices for a few days.

You may have 'Detox Symptoms' from the process of your body eliminating toxins, if they are too severe, stop for one day and start again with ½ dose. Symptoms may be nausea, headache etc. If you are allergic to sea weed or shell fish seek professional guidance on whether you can take chlorella or spirulina before you add them to juice, as they are sea algae.

2. Energy Lift

Ingredients

1 large carrot

$^1/_2$ avocado

$^1/_2$ beetroot

1 heaped tsp fresh parsley, chopped

1 tbsp barley grass powder or Spirulina or equivalent mixed green vegetable powder. Or simply use any green leafy vegetable.

2 turnip leaves

Ginger to taste

Optional: Barley grass or spirulina (organic only); any 'green' vegetable powder. Start with 1/3 tsp and increase if you wish to 1 tsp after you get used to the powerful taste of this smoothie.

• Ideally drink at your most tired time of the day.

If you find it too strong then water it down a little and sip it over 15 minutes.

3. Anemia Protection

Ingredients

2 sprigs parsley

2 leaves spinach /silver beet

3 prunes (remove the seeds)

$^1/_2$ cup blackberries or blue berries

$^1/_2$ raw beetroot

$^1/_2$ tsp vitamin C powder

Any sprouts

Note: if you feel nauseas after drinking the juice, it's because its too concentrated. Water it down to dilute, and sip it slowly.

Vegetable Juice Crystals/Powder

For those people who are too busy, can't be bothered with juicing or don't have a juicer, modern day technology has given us a quick, convenient method - Vegetable Juice crystals/powders (there are different varieties found in health stores and multi level marketing).

Simply add the carrot, barley grass and beetroot crystals/powder to water and drink. They still contain most of the natural goodness - it's all in the processing technique - and they often come with the advantage of the vegetables being grown organically.

(All available through my clinic or web site)

Brown Rice - Wholegrain Only!

- White rice is a perfect example of how food processing transforms a nutrient rich, high fiber food into a nutrient deficient imitation of its original self.

- Brown rice helps to balance blood sugar insulin and glucose, inhibits cholesterol synthesis and promotes good bowel health. Rice bran can help prevent Calcium from forming kidney stones.

- For those people doing Daniel's Diet, one of the great benefits of brown rice is that it will fill the stomach. There's no need to go hungry. It's what I call a neutral food, it's not acidic to your system, it's a good source of protein and soluble fiber, and can be eaten either sweet or savory.

- Brown rice though is not a complete protein; it doesn't contain all the necessary amino acids. However, when mixed with nuts and legumes that do include the missing nutrients, rice can become a complete protein meal. Cooked brown rice averages 5-7 grams of protein per cup.

- Basmati is high-amylose rice with a low glycemic index (sugar) rating therefore offering a healthy second option for those people who don't like brown rice.

"Can laborers and athletes be vegetarians?"

I often hear people say, "I can't eat just vegetables – I work too hard!" "I have a heavy training schedule for my sport. I must have meat protein, carbohydrates and lots of it."

That excuse doesn't hold any value these days. There are vegetarians in nearly every sporting activity and work place. From weight lifters to marathon runners, iron man athletes, footballers, and laborers - you name it. These people will tell you they have as much and probably more endurance and stamina than meat eaters [6]. However, you must fully understand how to get whole protein from your natural foods.

What's In Your Vegetables?
Most vegetables contain about 1-2 grams of protein per ounce. Cooked beans average about 7-8 grams per half cup. Seeds and nuts contain on average 4-8 grams of protein per quarter cup.

- Asparagus - Iron, Calcium, Folate, Beta Carotene, Bioflavonoid, Vitamin B's & C, Chlorophyll, Zinc
- Beans - Zinc, Potassium, Calcium, vitamin A, B's & C, Magnesium, Pectin, Chlorophyll
- Beetroot - (Beets) - Niacin, Calcium, Copper, Iron, Magnesium, Manganese, Phosphorous, Potassium, Zinc, Vitamins A, B1, B2, B5, B6, B9, B12 & C, trace elements. Also small quantities of: Tryptophan, Threonine, Isoleucine, Leucine, Lysine, Methionine, Cysteine, Phenylalanine, Tyrosine, Valine, Arginine, Histidine, Alanine, Aspartic acid, Glutamic acid, Glycine, Proline, Serine
- Broccoli - One of the top nutritious vegetables, Calcium, Vitamin C, B5 E & K, Beta-carotene, Folate, Magnesium, Bioflavonoid, Sulphur compounds, Iron, Chlorophyll and Hydroxycinnamic acids
- Cabbage - Calcium, Folate, Sulphur, Iron, Zinc, Bioflavonoid, Selenium, Vitamin B5, C & E
- Carrots - Beta Carotene, Calcium, Potassium, Bioflavonoid, Iron, Magnesium.
- Cauliflower - Potassium, Folate, Calcium, Magnesium, Vitamin B5 & E, Sulphur, Bioflavonoid
- Celery - Sodium, Calcium, Magnesium, Potassium, Sulphur, Bi-

oflavonoid, Vitamin C
- Chick Peas - Calcium, Magnesium
- Corn - Iron, Magnesium, Calcium, Vitamin A & B
- Cucumber - Potassium, Sulphur, Phosphorous, Calcium, Manganese, Vitamin C
- Dulse - Calcium, Folate, Bioflavonoid, Potassium, Beta-carotene, Vitamin C & E, Magnesium, Manganese, Iodine.
- Garlic - Calcium, Magnesium, Selenium, Zinc, Potassium, Manganese, Iodine, Vitamin C, Anti-microbial agents
- Capsicum (Bell Peppers) - Bioflavonoid, Magnesium, Vitamin C, Potassium
- Greens leafy Vegetables - Chlorophyll, Calcium, Folate, Magnesium, Iron, Magnesium, Bioflavonoid, Copper, Potassium, and Vitamin E & K, Cobalt
- Kale - Calcium, Magnesium, Bioflavonoid, Vitamin C & E, Potassium, Folate, Manganese, Copper, Iron, Sulphur, Chlorophyll, fibre.
- Kelp - Iodine, Calcium, Manganese, Silica, Selenium
- Legumes - Chloride, Copper, Manganese, Molybdenum, Niacin, Phosphorus, Calcium, Vitamin B1, B2, B3, B5, B6 & B17, Potassium, Iron, Chlorine, Magnesium, Zinc, Folate
- Millet - Potassium, Vitamin B17, Magnesium
- Parsley - Iron, Calcium, Vitamin C, Bioflavonoid, Beta-carotene, Magnesium
- Parsnip - Beta Carotene, Vitamin A, Magnesium, Silica
- Potatoes - Potassium, Sodium, Calcium, Magnesium, Manganese, Copper,
- Soybeans - Calcium, Chloride, Vitamin K, Phosphorus, Iron
- Spinach - High in Iron, Calcium, Riboflavin, Potassium, Vitamin A
- Sweet Potatoes - Beta Carotene, Vitamin C & E, Calcium, Magnesium
- Turnip - Calcium, Selenium, Potassium

Add Some Taste to Your Recipes

Pungent, spicy tastes or 'hot' flavours contain essential oils (not called 'essential' for nothing) and are high in antioxidants. Foods include garlic, peppers, onions, chillies, ginger, mustard, rosemary, thyme, horseradish, cloves, cumin, oregano and basil. These foods are great taste enhancers and at the same time have very powerful healing and prevention properties.

Astringent foods give that grimacing effect on our mucus membranes (try eating a lemon and you will know what I mean). Other more gentle tasting ones are lentils, apples, asparagus, cucumbers, spinach, green and black tea, berries and artichokes. Once again, the taste is a result of certain phytochemicals and nutrients that are specific to each plant and the healing properties they contain.

Bitter foods are that way for a purpose—to balance the diet with specific nutrients and prevent taste buds being perverted to craving sweet-tasting foods. Examples are mostly the 'greens' and edible herbs, like cumin, coriander, dill, rhubarb, saffron, fenugreek and aloe Vera. These herbs and medicinal ones are bitter because of their high concentration of phytochemicals, which contain the healing factors. Bitter greens help cleanse the liver and gallbladder. Parsley is not only a garnish on your plate that makes it look good, it helps cleanse and support the kidneys.

Your taste buds will change when you start including all these varieties of food in your daily diet and this program will give you the perfect start. Not only will it help you avoid sugary foods in the future, but it will help you enjoy the flavours of the wonderful natural foods.

The Importance of Water

Tap water is now well documented as being full of added chemicals (in most countries). Filled with fluoride, chlorine and environmental toxins, tap water can be considered detrimental to our health. For these reasons using some form of water purifier, either filtering or distilling, should be given very serious consideration.

When it comes to buying a filter, bear in mind that usually the most expensive ones are the best; however its money well spent. Just make sure to change the filters regularly. Also insist on a written guarantee stating it actually does filter out everything you want it to i.e. copper, lead, cadmium, fluoride, chlorine etc.

There are lots of different purifiers and distillers available. So do your homework before handing over the money, check with a reputable distributor and purchase one you can afford. Drinking clean water is another of the essential ingredients for long-term good health.

In general I find that people, especially those under the age of 30, are drinking less and less water. Instead they are turning to soda, processed fruit juices, tea, coffee, flavored milks and the like, for their fluids. This is because their bodies simply don't like the ingredients in the water (whether they consciously know it or not). Water was made for drinking. Substitutes are full of additives and harmful chemicals, they wear away insidiously at the body's metabolism, weakening it and creating a toxic overload. They are also a contributing factor to overloaded kidneys, causing fluid retention and a slowed down elimination process. If you suffer from fluid retention you must increase your water intake to eventually get rid of the excess fluid – don't cut down, as some people tend to do.

Large amounts of water must be consumed to help break up the fat cells that clump together. Research shows that eight to ten glasses (one to two quarts) of clean water should be consumed each day. This amount should not include other beverages especially since many of them (fruit and vegetable juices, coffee, tea and milk for example) are considered to be foods, not drinks. Water is also best drunk between meals, so as not to water down your digestive juices.

Whilst researching Chronic Fatigue Syndrome in the 80's I surveyed 300 people in Western Australia, and found the following results:
- 80% strongly disliked drinking the local tap water
- 15% were not concerned either way
- 5% actually thought it was fine

Many of those interviewed, mentioned how pure water is much sweeter and more palatable than standard tap water. I personally can tell pure water from tap in the first sip and sometimes even before by the smell of the Chlorine.

Purified tap water is recommended for this diet and bottled spring water is allowable. Squeezing a few drops of freshly squeezed lemon juice in the water adds some flavor and is also beneficial. Lemon aids the gastro intestinal tract, helps ward off bad bacteria and helps regulate the body's acid/alkaline balance. It also contains minerals and vitamins.

Green and herbal teas, (chamomile, peppermint and dandelion for example) made with clean water are excellent for the body. Anyone suffering from sugar cravings can add a quarter of a teaspoon of unprocessed honey or a small amount of Stevia to the drink. A little honey is reluctantly allowed – but don't overdo it.

Supplements
Probiotic:
Lactobacillus & Bifidobacterium (Optional). It's a great idea while cleansing our system to re–supply our intestinal area with natural flora like Lactobacillus, Acidophilus & Bifidobacteria. Don't be put off by the long names, they are the friendly bacteria naturally found in the bowel and intestines. These floras (called Probiotic) need to be regularly replenished because they are often destroyed through our modern lifestyles and the overuse of antibiotics. These bacteria are available in natural yogurt, but because of the high doses necessary to clinically replenish the gut, I strongly suggest using a professional supplement. Taking any less would simply not be enough. Also yogurt, being dairy, is not recommended on this diet. There are many strains of probiotics available, on this program simply use a good quality multi strain.

Fermented foods:
Fermented foods are called a pre-biotic which means it helps your tummy produce its own good bacteria. So adding fermented foods to this

diet plan would be an excellent idea. Cultured or fermented foods have a very long history in virtually all ancient diets (and would have been around in Daniels time), and have been known for their health benefits. It's the fermentation process that makes it such a great way to generate good healthy gut probiotic bacteria. Eating about a quarter to half a cup (2 to 4 oz) of fermented vegetables daily is all that is required. Examples are Sauerkraut, Kombucha, Kefir (dairy free), Kimchi, Natto and Tempeh.

PART TWO

HEALTHY IN BODY, SPIRIT & SOUL

CHAPTER ELEVEN

BODY, SOUL & SPIRIT

Each of us exists as a three part being. We are each a spirit encompassed in a body with a soul that gives us our emotions, personality and thoughts. These three parts are integral to our well-being and it is vital that we all understand the three-way connection between body, spirit and soul. I just want to clarify the word 'soul' because its meaning can vary in different cultures. When I talk about the soul in this book I refer to it in the context of our personality, emotions, **free will** and mind. So when I speak of body, spirit and soul it is the same as saying body, spirit and mind.

The Physical Realm

When God created us it was so that we could live in both the spiritual and the physical world. The Biblical viewpoint is that God created both the spiritual and the physical world for our benefit and enjoyment. Full enjoyment however, depends on us firstly understanding the spiritual side of our lives and following the principles or laws that govern both realms.

The human body is to be regarded as a dwelling place or home of the Holy Spirit. (1 Corinthians. 6:19-20) Therefore, it is important for us to flow and harmonize with laws that keep our bodies - the temples of the Holy Spirit - healthy.

Even those people who consider themselves to be spiritual must realize that the physical laws cannot be neglected, no matter how spiritual the person may be. Furthermore, those who consider themselves more on a physical plain must learn to understand the importance of the laws relating to the spiritual realm. Despite this need for balance among our three parts, mankind has always swayed to extremes. In the context of this book, the extreme is indulging in all the pleasures of the physical side (or flesh), becoming sensual and body-controlled. This is why we have a society that demands everything be instant – fast food, fast service, multiple sex partners, constant adrenaline rushes, and instant excitement or entertainment. A 'quick fix', instant gratification mentality is continually in need of fulfillment. Modern day society can also be selfish and very 'me' focused. This way of thinking and living is created because our physical nature is ruling our spiritual side. This is something that is in direct opposition to the original plan made for us. Our spirit as a Christian believer should be in control of our physical body, including our thinking. If we can only get this aspect of our nature into balance with the other parts of ourselves, then true health, healing, peace and prosperity will flourish.

A Healthy Body

By adopting *The Daniels Way to Weight Loss* and Renewed Energy it is possible to obtain and maintain a healthy body. Regular rest/sleep, holidays, exercise and a proper diet are keys to achieving this. But it's also important to understand what God's expectation of us is, in regard to our bodies. In essence we need to be a good steward of our body. The Bible says that it's up to us to look after our bodies, it's a task expected of each one of us (stewardship).

Everyone can choose to eat whatever he or she likes, but in doing so are you being unwise and being brought under that food's power? Are you being dictated to by cravings and addictions and selfish desires?

Are you sick because of a poor diet or lifestyle?

Paul (the Apostle), addressed the concept of freedom of choice in 1 Corinthians 6:12 *"All things are lawful for me, but all things are not helpful. All things are lawful for me, but I will not be brought under the power of any...For you were brought with a price; therefore glorify God in your body and in your spirit, which are*

God's."

We only have one body and one opportunity to be a good steward of that which God has given us. Taking that into consideration, and the fact that everybody wants to enjoy longevity and quality of life whilst on planet earth, isn't it worth the effort of making the changes to ensure good health?

My favorite saying when I am teaching at Churches is this; "Are you working with Jesus for your healing or against Him?" Meaning, are you doing your part in being healthy, are you following Gods Natural Health Principles and living a healthy lifestyle? If you do your part God will do the rest.

A Healthy Spirit

When God first created mankind He breathed His spirit into us and we became a living soul. (Genesis 2:7) In fact, without our spirit the inner person, or real you would have no life. The book of James 2:26, tells us that the *"body without the spirit is dead."*

It's interesting to note that our spirit and soul were designed to rule over and control our body. As I have already mentioned, we often see the reverse. A weak spirit produces a weak mind and subsequently a weak body. The laws of health in the spirit realm all relate to laws that feed, train and strengthen the spirit man. The purpose of these laws is to produce a healthy and strong spirit. A strong, vibrant spirit produces health in the soul and in the body. It should then become clear that one of the keys to great health is to learn the secret of keeping our spirits healthy.

In Proverbs 20:27 it says our human spirit *"is the lamp of the Lord."* This tells us that our human spirit is our contact point when it comes to communicating with God, because He is a Spirit.

Therefore, it's vital to become and stay, spiritually alive. So because our human spirit is our main connection with God, and because it's eternal, it stands to reason that this aspect of us needs the most nurturing.

If you are spiritually healthy you have peace, resistance to stress and anxiety, inner strength, contentment and satisfaction in life. A vibrant (healthy) spirit produces (or lays the foundation) for health in the soul and in the physical body. *"A broken spirit dries the bones."* (Proverbs 17:22) *"The spirit of a man will sustain him in sickness but who can bear a broken spirit?"* (Proverbs 18:14)

How often do we see very rich and beautiful people (who seemingly 'have it all'), who are actually really unhappy or unfulfilled in life? People will try all sorts of extreme things such as drugs to 'fix' themselves, sadly only to feel some distorted happiness. Others have multiple sexual partners to find fulfillment in life. The answer in most of these cases is to find spiritual wholeness.

One of the keys to true, divine health is learning the secret of keeping our spirit healthy. God does have a Health Plan and its essence is, "Sow good nourishment to all three parts of your being" by using:

1. Food from God's garden and a healthy, moderate lifestyle for your **body**.
2. A positive mental attitude and regular reading of The Word of God for your **soul**.
3. The opportunity to communicate personally with God through times of prayer, meditation, reading from Scripture (John 6:63) and positive fellowship with like-minded people to feed your **spirit**.

The common denominator is that all 3 parts have to be fed the right food, whether it might be spiritual, intellectual or physical food because if you feed any one of them with wrong things it will eventually cause a problem.

We take our spirit everywhere we physically go and if we have a headache or feel sick or tired in any way it will affect our spirit because our spirit is found in our body.

I am talking about your human spirit here, but what about the Holy Spirit, our spiritual connection to God?

When we spiritually connect to God's Holy Spirit we become spiritually alive or reborn. This is our own spiritual awakening. It isn't something 'weird' but something to enjoy and be eternally grateful for, accept it as the wonderfully spiritual and fulfilling experience it is.

The Soul Realm (the Emotions, the Personality and the Mind)
There are sicknesses of the soul just as there are sicknesses of the body. But, because there are no measurements to define what the optimum healthy soul should be like, they cannot be easily classified. However, the Bible does make reference to some classifications on this subject. A healthy soul is full of love, joy, hope, faith and peace, with a positive approach to life. An unhealthy soul is the opposite; it's filled with hate, selfishness, disbelief, unforgiveness, sorrow, depression and fear.

An unhealthy soul will have self talk like:
- "I can't." • "It'll never work."
- "I don't believe in God." • "I don't care."
- "It's someone else's fault." • "I'll never be happy."
- "I can forgive but I won't forget."
- "If God is real (or cares) – why is there so much suffering in the world?"
- "God doesn't listen – He won't answer my prayers."

A healthy soul will definitely lead to a healthy body and vice versa.
I have noticed over my years as a practitioner the many links between illness and an unhealthy soul
This link does not relate to everybody suffering from the symptoms listed below, but I have found that it relates to many people I meet. In today's terminology the sicknesses might be referred to as psychosomatic.

The symptoms and links include: from my clinical and ministerial observations:
- Poor eyesight is linked with people carrying sorrow in their heart and mind for too long. (Psalm 6:7)

- Bowel and Intestinal problems are linked with holding onto unhappiness, unfulfilment and lack of achievement in life and living with past regrets; the accumulation of stress.
- Excessive appetite is linked with a need for self-protection, escapism; a feeling of fear, that things are too hard to face; a sense of being overwhelmed by everyday life.
- Asthma is linked with fear and anxiety; suppressed emotions.
- Anxiety and fear can also be connected to IBS (irritable bowel syndrome), heart palpitations.
- Some Cancer may be linked with lack of forgiveness and stored up hatred; deep hurts and grief eating away internally; lack of hope, or excess pride.
- Senility may be linked with escapism, reverting back to the safety of childhood, a form of controlling and demanding attention, especially from family.
- Arthritis may be linked with resentment and lack of forgiveness.
- Heart disease is often linked with stress and depression.

Because some sicknesses are soul related, they do not respond for long, if at all to normal treatments. These people need spiritual help/counseling and healing, physical supplements and diet will help but it's secondary. The first step to helping these situations is to (a) recognize it (b) talk to a person who is a strong Christian and get prayer.

Jesus ministered forgiveness to the paralyzed man before He prayed for physical healing. (Mark 2:5) There are many modern day churches and counseling services that will pray for and nurture those who need help.

A healthy soul is full of love, joy, hope, faith and peace

Lord Shaftesbury, the evangelical social reformer, told a Social Service Congress at Liverpool, England, in 1859, *"When people say we should think more of the soul and less of the body, my answer is that the same God who made the soul made the body also...I maintain that God is worshiped not only by the spiritual but also by the material creation. Our bodies, the temple of the Holy Ghost, ought not to be corrupted by preventable disease, degraded by avoidable filth, and disabled for his service by unnecessary suffering."*

Understanding the Character of God for Our Health and Wellbeing

It is God's perfect will that all of us, His children, enjoy perfect health. It's wonderful to be healed of a problem but even more wonderful to be in good health and never get the sickness in the first place. Health and healing are a part of the Covenant promised to all believers forever, and that includes you and me. (Exodus 23:25)

However, as with any agreement there are conditions:

- IF you listen carefully
- IF you do what is morally right
- IF you pay attention to His commands
- IF you keep all His decrees

These laws or principles are not designed to make life hard – but to protect us and bless us with health, healing and prosperity. God gave us laws, teachings and guidelines to follow in the spiritual realm, but He also gave us teachings for use in the practical realm.

God has a holistic health plan for us to discover and follow today. A plan for our body, soul and spirit. But to reach perfect health we must first learn and understand these rules. Then 'if' we listen and obey them, health and healing is yours to expect and enjoy. Being in good health is not an accident, nor is it something to be taken for granted or only appreciated when you get sick. Health needs to be maintained. It's a product of our own individual choices. Obeying God's laws maintains harmony in all aspects of mind, body and spirit. Neglecting just one of these areas can cause disruption to the equilibrium of our being.

It is a common experience that what goes on in either the spirit, the soul or the body will affect the other two parts. Our spirit, soul and body are intricately intertwined and only separate at death. For instance:

Physical tiredness affects our mental ability to concentrate and to make decisions. It can also make us irritable, impatient, emotionally vulnerable and perhaps a little selfish.

Consistent destructive thoughts of unforgiveness, bitterness, anger or depression can eventually cause physical diseases, even though it originates in the soul.

A lack of spiritual tranquility or fulfillment stirs unrest in the soul. It can cause a feeling of heaviness, unhappiness and of never being fully content with life. Manifesting itself in the search for spiritual fulfillment through witchcraft, new age occultism, drugs, excess alcohol, sexual promiscuity, love of money, adrenaline cravings and belief in false gods. All these phenomena may seem exciting in the short term but, in the long term, they lead to a deeper unfulfillment, unhappiness, bad luck, emptiness and destruction. Since we are all born with a human spirit, everyone whether they know it or not is seeking a fulfillment of this spiritual self.

I personally have searched for this fulfillment in most of the areas listed above, and finally I was introduced to Jesus as the true spiritual connection, applied His principles to my life and it's been the best thing to ever happen to me. It's brought me fulfillment to my life and peace to my soul. Some people may also wonder why I quote the Bible. It's because it is the only book that gives answers for the beginning of life, what to do in the middle and what happens at the end. It gives the answers to all the whys and wherefores of life. It also puts loving your neighbor and yourself as its top priority. I don't know about you but I want to know why I am on earth and where I am going after I leave.

Whilst the spirit realm is the predominant influence of all three parts of our being, the influence of the soul and body must not be underestimated.

The power of food and physical hunger should never be overlooked. Many people today are making unwise, hasty decisions based upon their appetites and cravings, and will suffer the consequences. A man in the Bible, Esau, gave away his family inheritance for a meal of red lentil stew because he was hungry. (Genesis 25:29-34)

The secret to health and fulfillment is a simple one. Understand the balance between spirit, soul and body and feed all three with the right ingredients. Do not neglect one or any other.

PART THREE

THE DIET

CHAPTER TWELVE

MAKING DANIEL'S DIET EASIER

Before starting the Daniel's Diet I would advise that everybody give themselves the best chance of successfully and easily completing the diet by:

- Avoiding all caffeine products (foods and drinks)
- Removing as much sugar as possible from their diet
- Significantly cutting down on white flour products
- Cutting down on all dairy products
- Stop alcohol
- Increasing water intake to two quarts daily
- Sourcing the appropriate herbs and vitamins you may need and begin taking them

Why? The reason I advise this is because these foods often give strong withdrawal reactions such as headaches, nausea, cravings, emotional fragility, etc. Other foods or drinks may also be causing the toxic reactions but generally the effects are not as strong as those caused by caffeine, white flour, dairy foods and sugar. Dependant on each person's level of toxicity or addiction withdrawal symptoms may last for one to four days and vary in severity. In other words the worse you feel in the first few days the more toxic are your tissues and you are feeling the 'detox' working. Don't give up. The moment you eat something not on the diet, the unpleasant symptoms may disappear because you have STOPED the detoxification process. Eliminating harmful foods before starting Daniel's Diet means that the progress and benefits of the diet will appear more quickly. In other words, by cutting out these foods before the commencement, the diet will be easier to adhere to.

By approximately Day 3, everyone should generally start to feel internally 'cleaner' and better. The longer the detoxification or withdrawal symptoms take to work through, the more toxins there were in the body and the more necessary this program was.

Many people who have completed this diet have commented that they were shocked or surprised at the strength of the withdrawal symptoms they experienced and how it made them acutely aware of just how toxic their body was. Their realizations that it was obviously caffeine, sugar or another food causing the worst symptoms only made them more determined to cut out that particular culprit food from their diet in the future

Case History
Most extreme 'withdrawal' reaction recorded so far!

'My Last Will and Testament!'
Beryl's Story'; *she was very sick and her symptoms were numerous; Chronic Fatigue Syndrome, coughing every morning until she was close to blacking out, feeling pressure around her heart, depression, her joints were full of arthritic pain, she was wearing a splint on her arm because of the pain in her wrist and hands (she was scheduled to have an operation on her arm and wrist, but was putting it off because she would never be able to play the piano again). She said 'she felt like a truck had run over her' because her muscles were so sore all over. Beryl also had reflux and digestive problems. She was 33 pounds (15 kg) overweight and her body had a lot of fluid retention, 'I was puffy all over' she said!*

Consultation with me:

Her diet was poor and predominately refined carbohydrates. So I made up a No list of the things that were harming her most;
- Coffee (she was having 10 cups per day with 2 sugars and milk).
- All dairy
- White flour products (all gluten foods)

- Alcohol
- Chocolate and all sugar/sweets

I sent her home to prepare for the diet with a mixture of herb supplements.

Beryl being a strong willed and determined person went home and straight onto the diet with no pre diet preparation (her choice and not wise, preparation is important).

On day three of the diet she was feeling so bad from withdrawals, she was bed ridden and called her family to the bed side to write out her ' last Will & Testament' as she thought/felt she was going to die! I admire that she stayed on the diet plan all the way through.

The withdrawals lasted for 7 days. She said was willing to go through the withdrawals with her families support, because she was determined to get well as she was so fed up and tired of feeling sick in the first place. She believed God wanted her healthy and that she had to do her part in achieving this.

The Good News;
She comes back in to my clinic 3 weeks later —'a new woman'.

When she told me (in her feisty, dry sense of humor style) about writing out her 'Will' and how extreme the withdrawals affected her — I (and her daughter) had the biggest belly laugh because it was so extreme and she was now so obviously better for it and full of health and vitality, compared to the first time I spoke with her.

Her cough had gone completely; she was off her reflux medication as there was no longer any need for it; she felt no heart pressure, no need for the splint on her arm (no need for any operation), lost 11pounds (5 kg) in weight; had lots more energy and less pain. In fact she was considering going back to work in the family's business.

One month later on her third consult, it was hard to believe I was talking to the same women I first met less than 2 months ago. She was happy, laughing and joking and just full of life.

She had lost 17.6 pounds (8 Kg) and all the puffiness (fluid retention) had gone. She said 'I now wake up in the morning wanting to get out of bed and enjoy life , instead of wanting to pull the sheets over my head and not face the day like I felt before'.

Beryl is now Daniel's Way biggest fan (and a friend of mine for life she says) and largest individual purchaser of my books. People are continually saying to her 'wow you have lost weight and whatever you are on I want some', (including her pastor's wife). She now buys bulk amounts of this book every time I see her and gives them away to people, to help them, because it helped her so much. (I have added her testimony after the first print of this book as it was so profound)

Caution: if you have a severe reaction when doing a fast or detox, it's wise to stop and do the recommended pre diet preparation. Then start again when your body is read, doing it more slowly. The results are worth it.

Pre-Diet Plan

Daniel's Diet gives everyone the opportunity to recognize and break bad habits and addictions.

Some people may choose to start the diet straight away, regardless of the withdrawal symptoms. However, it's using wisdom to follow the pre- diet plan to make it less traumatic on your body. To help recognize danger foods, I recommend working to a plan.

I suggest a commitment plan for two weeks. It is your choice however as I know a lot of people don't want to wait and that is ok too.

Week 1 - Pre-Diet:

Ask yourself the question, "What are the most common and therefore harmful foods that I am eating?"

Just pick two to start with.

Write them down.

_____

_____

Now choose not to eat them.

YOUR JOURNEY HAS BEGUN. Make it an enjoyable life changing experience.

You may have to admit that chocolates, chips/crisps, fries or breads are not good for you, but remember changing some of your old self-talk will help too.

"Death and life are in the power of the tongue, and those who love it will eat its fruit." (Pro.18: 21 NKJV)

We all have to live with the consequences of everything we do. There is a consequence for every decision we make. What you decide to eat today will have a consequence tomorrow. It's up to you whether you choose life or death.

Now you have committed to stopping some of the danger foods, begin to focus on all the foods this diet recommends you to eat rather than those you need to avoid.

Use affirmations like:
- "Salad and fruits are my favorite foods."
- "I choose to stop eating sugary and fatty foods."
- "I choose to enjoy eating vegetables."

Some people will be ready at this stage to start Daniel's Diet. Others may choose to prepare for another week. Both are fine. Everyone is an individual, start when you are ready.

Week 2:

Look at your list of foods and decide what your next two danger foods are?

_____

_____

Now choose not to eat them.

By simply not eating these items, you have started the pre-diet plan for eliminating the danger foods. That means you are now eating less of the foods that were causing cravings and weight problems. Well done!

When it comes to breaking the habits and addiction, some of the culprit foods may take longer than others to overcome. Don't let this be a concern, it doesn't matter how long it takes, what's important is that you are progressing towards your goals.

By this stage most people will be ready to start Daniel's Diet. Having recognized and overcome some of the addictive foods, successfully completing the 10 days should be much easier.

Don't fall back into the trap of justifying your addiction with negative self-talk.

Remember you are not under any old fashioned laws but are free to choose, so choose wisely, and choose to be healthy:
- "I choose to give up the foods that are harming me."
- "I choose to enjoy eating only healthy foods."
- "I choose to be healthy; I have the right to be healthy."

Over the years I have had many people give me excuses for not doing the diet; I have even had the Bible quoted at me. "The Bible says I can eat anything I want," they said, "so I will." My answer to this is, "The Bible says you can eat all things that are good, for food. NOT any and everything, and especially not the ones that you are addicted, or the ones that are harmful."

"Listen carefully to Me, and eat what is good." (Isaiah 55:2)

An excellent tongue in cheek statement I once heard a Preacher say was in answer to the question. "Will I still go to heaven," a young man asked, "if I eat lots of junk food?"

"Yes," replied the Preacher, "but you will go there a lot quicker."

It's not so much willpower that is needed, but knowing what is the right thing to do. That's why I go into details before revealing the diet. To succeed there must be the desire and choice to live a healthy, fit, long and prosperous life. The desire is enhanced by understanding why it's important to look after yourself, but YOU must want to do this diet.

"Test us for ten days," he said. *"Give us vegetables to eat and water to drink."* Daniel 1:12 (GNB)

"When the time was up they looked healthier and stronger than all those who had been eating the royal food." Daniel 1: 15

Pre-Diet Shopping List

You won't be surprised that vegetables and clean water are first on the shopping list. However, to make the diet more interesting there are lots of tasty foods to include.

It's wise to know what to shop for before starting the diet. This avoids the risk of being caught without any of the recommended foods on hand when you are hungry, lessening the chance of being tempted back to fast food, white bread and other unhealthy foods.

Anyone who has been eating the same way for many years, who then suddenly decides to make changes to their diet is bound to require some time for adjustment. To these people it may seem to take longer to shop and prepare meals, but this is only due to reading labels, thinking differently and changing habits. Given just a short period of time this new way of living and eating will become normal to you and subsequently as easy and as normal as what you were doing previously.

Cooking for health is taking advantage of basic, simple and natural foods, and putting them together into different and appetizing forms. Their natural flavors can then be further enhanced by the use of herbs and natural seasonings. If you do this, even a simple salad or vegetable dish tastes delicious. The trick is to make it look and taste great, something everyone can achieve with a little practice and effort.

The Good Food Kitchen

Essential utensils for the 'good food kitchen' include; stainless steel cookware, wooden chopping board, ceramic cook ware, a steamer or steamer inserts; a blender or food processor and a suitable vegetable shredder. A juicer, pressure cooker or crock-pot for dried beans, peas and lentils are also valuable assets. A Spirooli machine or Slicer is a great tool for making noodles with vegetables. The Spirooli makes thick noodle cuts and is perfect for zucchini spaghetti/noodles recipes – see the salad recipes in this book for a yummy recipe using this easy to use slicer.

As are a wok, rice steamer, bake ware and wooden spoons for delicate mixes, such as sauces. No aluminum or copper cook ware.

It is helpful to find a thriving health store in your area. There are many organic vegetable suppliers around and if you are having trouble locating one ask your naturopath or at your local health store. The people involved in natural health usually have a network to draw from.

Remember all natural fruit and vegetables are allowed – use variety and make your plate the color of a rainbow. I encourage you to create new ideas and use things you have not used before.

The food list

It is helpful to find a thriving health store in your area. There are many organic vegetable suppliers around and if you are having trouble locating one ask your naturopath or at your local health store. The people involved in natural health usually have a network to draw from.

There are also vegetarian cooking classes in most towns or cities for those who wish to learn more in that field.

Here is a list of the necessary products for this diet. I was able to get them all from my local health store.

- Dried beans, all varieties: navy, black-eyed, green, broad, etc
- Red and green lentils, split peas
- Organic Tamari; an all natural, all purpose, wheat free soy sauce. It enhances the taste of salads, vegetable dishes, brown rice dishes and potatoes.
- Organic Herb seasoning - It comes in different varieties, including one for soup stock. They can be found in most local supermarkets.
- Celtic sea salt (or Himalayan salt) and cayenne pepper

- Herbal soup stock - No MSG or hydrolyzed vegetable protein
- Garlic and dried, organic herbs
- Brown rice or Basmati
- Shitake. and Reishi mushrooms. These mushrooms are immune boosters.
- Stevia for a sweetener. Do not use chemical (diet) sweeteners e.g. saccharin and aspartame.
- Lots of fresh fruits and vegetables. Variety is important especially from the 'cruciferous' vegetables: broccoli, cabbage, Brussels sprouts and cauliflower. One or more of these should be eaten every day. Use fresh where at all possible, frozen is the second choice. Avoid canned and packet foods.
- Natural soap without chemicals and with natural fragrance
- Natural toothpaste and deodorant (containing no aluminum).
- * White vinegar – to wash your fruit and vegetables with. Or ask at your local health shop for a natural product to help wash off the toxins. White vinegar is very good for a house hold cleaner. Use it for cleaning floors, showers, toilets and burnt pots.
- Miso (kome or genmal) is a fermented soy product with sea salt, rice and water. It's a great addition to flavor soups and vegetable casseroles.
- Soup stock. Find a vegetable-only one which can be found in most supermarkets or health stores.
- Sun-dried tomatoes and fruit. Dried fruit often contains sulphur to enhance the color of the dried product. Seek organic sundried fruit, which is also sulphur- free. This is especially important if you experience any respiratory challenges such as asthma.
- Prunes.
- Corn thins/rice wafers. They must be made of only corn or rice, and water.
- Dried, organic herbs.
- Organic Apple Cider Vinegar, in glass bottles. The only vinegar allowed on this diet.

- Herbal teas; Chamomile, peppermint, fennel, dandelion and green tea;
- Braggs ™ Liquid Amino. This is a healthy, natural flavor-enhancer worth experimenting with. It's made from soy and contains amino acids that are essential to our health. Everyone, especially vegetarians, would be wise to include this in their long-term diet.
- Soups. Try making up a large pot of vegetable soup using the allowed ingredients, then freeze or refrigerate it to create quick meals.
- Try adding seaweed to your foods.
- Stir-fry. You'll find a wonderful selection of frozen stir-fry vegetable mixes in the freezer section of your local supermarket. Make sure you choose the ones with no added sauces. The store will also have bags of prepared raw stir-fry vegetables in the fresh food section, though you will probably have to add more colours yourself. Choose fresh foods where possible, however frozen are good as a second choice and for convenience. To avoid plastic contamination, I recommend you mix your own from the loose choices available, i.e. bag up your own.
- Lentils. Buy a good selection of beans (black eyed, haricot, kidney, chick peas, etc.) and cook about ¼ of them prior to starting the diet, or on the first day. These can be kept in the refrigerator, then added to salads or soups each day to create variety, and to act as a filler

Dried herbs and spices
- Bay leaves
- Cayenne (red) pepper
- Chia
- Chili powder
- Cinnamon sticks
- Cloves
- Cumin

- Curry powder
- Dried Herbs
- Garlic
- Ground cinnamon
- Ground coriander
- Ground or fresh ginger
- Ground nutmeg
- Masala
- Marjoram
- Mustard Powder
- Onion
- Paprika
- Peppercorns green and black
- Sesame Seeds
- Turmeric

Nuts & seeds (unsalted) and dried fruit
- Almonds (blanched or whole)
- Hazelnuts
- Pecans
- Pine nuts
- Prunes
- Sun-dried tomatoes
- Walnuts
- Brazil
- Cashews
- Pumpkin seeds
- Sunflower seeds
- Sesame seeds
- Chia seeds

Dried fruit often contains sulphur to enhance the color of the dried product. Seek organic sun-dried fruit, which is also sulphur- free. This is especially important if you experience any respiratory challenges such as asthma.

No peanuts and limit the cashews.

Stir-fry

You'll find a wonderful selection of frozen stir-fry vegetable mixes in the freezer section of your local supermarket. Make sure you choose the ones with no added sauces. The store will also have bags of prepared raw stir-fry vegetables in the fresh food section, add more colours yourself if needed. Choose fresh foods where possible, however frozen are good as a second choice and for convenience. To avoid plastic contamination, I recommend you mix your own from the loose choices available, i.e. bag up your own.

Please note: Eat to your body size and appetite. E.g. some people may need rice and lentils every day to be able to feel full. Do not over eat.

CHAPTER THIRTEEN

THE DIET

L et's take a look at what you can and can't eat whilst on Daniel's Diet. This is one of the most profound - life changing and healthy diets I have seen in over 25 years as a health practitioner. I have the testimonies of myself and numerous others to prove it. The reason it is so beneficial and the results so fantastic is because you don't eat any of the man made processed, manufactured or adulterated foods. We get back to the basics of eating only natural, unprocessed foods. There is only one criterion "YOU HAVE TO DO IT". I encourage you take a step of faith & see what God will do!

NOT ALLOWED
Foods that are NOT Allowed on this Program

NO - Dairy food
This includes; any of the following ingredients added to foods: Milk solids, skim milk, milk protein, non milk fat solids, whey, casein, caseinate, lactose, sustagen, drinking chocolate (or equivalent).

This includes NO:
- Cow's milk
- Butter Ice cream
- Cheese
- Chocolate
- Cream Yoghurt
- Cream soups

- Mayonnaise Dairy based dips

Don't worry you will get adequate calcium from all the vegetables, seeds, nuts and fruits you are now eating.

NO - Wheat or other gluten grains
This includes NO:

- Bread
- Pastry
- Breakfast cereal
- Cereal/grain coffee (chicory is ok)
- Gravy
- Cake
- Sauce
- Pasta
- Biscuits/Crackers
- Cookies

(Refer to section on grain, *chapter 9*)

NO - Caffeine
This includes NO:

- Coffee
- Black tea
- Cola drinks
- Cocoa
- Decaffeinated coffee
- Energy drinks
- Flavored milk drinks or diet powders

(Refer to section on coffee/caffeine and tea, *chapter 9*)

NO - Fruit Juices
This includes NO:

- Fruit juices (shop bought or home-made); 100% fruit down to 25% (or lower).

NO - Yeast
This includes NO:

- Bread
- Yeast based spreads
- Vegemite
- Beer

NO - Sugar
This includes NO:
- Granulated sugar of ANY color (brown sugar is no different to white, its just colored)
- Artificial (diet) sweeteners
- Candy/sweets
- Breath fresheners or chewing gum (even if sugar free)

NO - Fried foods
This includes NO:
- Foods cooked in oil and foods soaked in oil to enable them to be baked (i.e. oven fries/chips)

NO - Chemicals
This includes NO:
- Artificial sweeteners
- Monosodium Glutamate (MSG)
- Artificial preservatives
- Artificial flavorings
- Colorings

NO - Sauces & spreads.
All shop bought ones, as these have too many additives and are mostly very acid.

NO - Gravies.
Most have flour (grain) base and chemicals additives

NO - Eggs

NO - White Rice

NO - Table Salt

NO - Alcohol

Limit Potatoes

Whilst these are a vegetable they should only be eaten in moderation. Potatoes tend to be over consumed in our society. They are a carbohydrate with a high Glycemic index, which means they can interfere in some people's ability to lose weight. If you do choose to eat them during this 10-day program eat them during the middle of the day and not in the evenings. This will lessen their affect on your weight loss. To benefit from the nutrients they contain bake or steam potatoes and eat them with their skins on.

Sweet potatoes come from an entirely differently family to the potato despite their name. They are very nutritious and can be eaten every second day, instead of ordinary potatoes.

NO - Microwave cooking

MY TOP 10 'BAD FOODS'

It's not that hard really! By simply recognizing the most 'dangerous' foods and avoiding them you can add years to your life and lose kilos off your weight!

1. French Fries, hot chips, potato wedges.
2. Soda/Soft Drinks (including most cordials)
3. Chocolate
4. Packet Chips/crisps
5. Doughnuts
6. Most white flour products, bread, biscuits/cookies, pizza, cakes, pasta, packet cereal, pastry
7. Instant Noodles
8. Packet (iced) dairy drinks e.g. coffee & chocolate
9. Ice cream and confectionary (candy)
10. Over-refined and heated oils like margarines, fried food and processed foods such as takeaways.

They can block the arteries and thicken the blood. These products contain trans-fatty acids, sometimes called hydrogenated fats, and are a notorious culprit in heart disease and cancer.

Ask yourself the question, "What are the most common foods that I am eating off this list (add to the list if you Want to; e.g. alcohol, candy/lollies, biscuits etc?" Write them down here:

_____

_____

_____

ALLOWED
This Ten Day Diet - **A Partial Fast**
This Diet Plan is different from most other diets in that it's a partial fast for a set amount of time. A complete fast requires eating no food. A partial fast on the other hand allows unlimited (with wisdom) amounts of specified food.

This principle of partial fasting can become a good short-term discipline and thereby a great help in the long-term goal of longevity of diet and weight control. Especially after harmful foods have been recognized and rejected. Fasting of any kind is an overlooked and underestimated principle in today's society.

Eat Only The Food from 'Gods Garden.'
The rule of thumb is to eat any edible food that grows naturally. Keep in mind that God designed these wonderful, tasty life giving foods.

I encourage you to eat lots of varieties of fruit and vegetables, seeds and nuts, along with, unrefined carbohydrates and vegetable protein. I do give examples of recipes in this book (however see my book Daniels Way Recipe Guide for more specific recipes to help you on this diet plan). I encourage you to keep it simple and as long as you eat the allowed foods and don't eat the 'bad' foods then you won't go wrong. In other words the recipes are available to help but feel free to make up your own vegetarian meals. The following are my suggestions to help some of your choices.

Vegetables

All vegetables should be eaten raw, steamed or baked. Avoid using margarine, butter or table salt on them. Instead try flavoring them with herbs or a little coarse textured Himalayan rock salt or Celtic (natural) salt, this should be grey in color because of the many trace minerals it contains. You can also use vegetable salt (ask at your health store where to source it from).

All vegetables, in any quantity, are allowed but especially:

• Beans	• Beets	• Broccoli
• Brussels Sprouts	• Cabbage	• Carrot
• Bell Peppers (Red)	• Cauliflower	• Celery
• Lentils	• Spinach	• Sprouts
• Pumpkin	• Sweet Potato	• Turnip

Aim at making rainbow salads by using several varieties of lettuce and vegetables that make up all the colors of the rainbow. Add avocado for its essential oils.

You can use fresh homemade vegetable sauces like – tomatoes, onions, garlic and herbs, mixed with water and slowly cooked at low temperatures. Spread this over steamed vegetables to enhance the flavor.

Ideas for Low – Glycaemic Vegetables

• Herbs & Spices	• Ginger
• Avocado	• Lettuce
• Alfalfa	• Leeks
• Asian Greens	• Mushrooms
• Asparagus	• Onions
• Bean Sprouts	• Parsley
• Green beans	• Cucumber
• Bok Choy	Pumpkin

- Broccoli
- Brussels Sprout
- Cabbage
- Salad Greens
- Capsicum
- Fennel
- Garlic
- Carrots
- Cauliflower
- Celery
- Chard

Radish
Rocket
Silver beet
Shallots
Eggplant
Squash
Spinach
Sprouts
Watercress
Zucchini
Collards

Nuts & Seeds
- Almonds
- Walnuts
- Sunflower Seeds

- Pine Nuts
- Pumpkin Seeds (Pepitas)
- Brazil

Ensure all nuts and seeds are fresh when they are purchased; this is more likely if they are purchased from a store with a high turnover. Nuts; if they taste bitter are probably rancid or stale and as such can create free radical toxins. No salted nuts and no peanuts (high allergy food).

Nuts and Seed Mix
No cashews (or maximum of 10). Use a standard 1 (small) cup measuring container and place a single layer of each of the following: almonds, walnuts or pecans, brazil nuts, pumpkin seeds, pine nuts and sunflower seeds. Pour mixture into a breakfast bowl and mix up. These are your 'between meals' snacks.

You don't have to eat it all in one day. If you're not hungry, keep some for the next day. Do not eat more than one cup of this mix per serve. If you feel any adverse affects after eating nuts, you would be advised to stop them entirely.

* If you are allergic to nuts – do not eat them.

All Fruit

I recommend everyone, except diabetics, to eat three to four different varieties of fruit per day. Eat one to two pieces at one sitting or consider having a fruit salad made up of half of four different fruits, apple, orange, pear and banana, for example. Whilst several pieces of fruit are allowed each day, fruit juices are to be avoided.

Be bold and experiment e.g. berries, melons, stone fruit, tropical, citrus, vine, apples and pears.

Rice – Brown or Basmati

Rice is an excellent filler to stave off hunger. Brown is first choice, although Basmati is acceptable because it has low GI. On this diet, one average sized bowl of cooked rice each or every second day is recommended. Try mixing garlic, onion, ginger, turmeric, cayenne or any natural herb with it to enhance the taste.

The following foods are permitted only once per day:
- Lentils - one cup
- Brown (daily) or Basmati rice (every second day is preferable) - one cup

Dandelion Coffee

Dandelion coffee - preferably organic - (sometimes called Dandelion Tea or Beverage) is the only form of coffee allowed. It is an excellent herbal substitute for caffeine and stimulates the liver, gall bladder and digestion. Check the labels – no lactose or sugars should be added and make sure it's a pure form of Dandelion.

Tea

Various herbal teas e.g. Chamomile, Peppermint, Fennel and Green Tea are allowed on this diet. Laxative herb teas are beneficial. Drink them plain or with a slice of lemon.

Water
To keep the body hydrated and to help flush out the toxins it's important to drink 1 to 2 quarts (two liters) of purified water a day. This amount should be on top of daily drinks of tea.

Sweeteners
Stevia, a natural herbal sweetener, purchased from health stores, are acceptable and safe to use. Small amounts of unprocessed honey or molasses may also be used to overcome any sugar cravings, but only if necessary and only in moderation. Do not use any other sweeteners.

My Top 10 'Miracle' Foods
- Broccoli
- Spinach
- Brussels sprouts
- Kale
- Prunes
- All berries – blue, black, raspberries, strawberries
- Tomatoes (cooked or raw)
- Orange-coloured foods – pumpkin and carrots
- Asparagus
- Sprouts (all raw sprouts)

It is worth noting that all these foods are alkaline in nature. The idea is to include all of them in your diet and to eat 3 or more of the fruits and 3 or more of the vegetables on a daily basis and eliminate as much as possible the sugary, white flour, fried and fatty foods from your lifestyle. Balancing your pH or acid – alkaline ratios is important for your health and weight loss.

The Top 2 'Miracle' Drinks
1. Water (1-2 litres daily)—which should be clean, i.e. purified/filtered. The average body loses about 2 quarts of water each day through normal elimination and perspiration/evaporation. This

must be replenished daily. This includes your cups of green tea or juices.

2. Green tea, with a squeeze of lemon. Green tea enhances abdominal fat loss. [1]

Meal Suggestions Whilst on Daniel's Diet
Golden rule: **Keep it simple**.

The idea is to make the ten days on the diet as easy and less time consuming as possible.

Those who have other people to cook for you will need to work a plan that only you know will work in your individual situation. One suggestion is by keeping it simple, you will find the diet less intrusive on your normal cooking for the family. By increasing your serving size of vegetables, and serving your food before there is any addition of additives (flavorings, sauces, gravies, mayonnaise, etc) and eating no meat, you can continue to cook for the family as you normally would.

Salad vegetables
All major supermarkets have pre-packaged salad greens and salad mixes. This is an excellent way of getting a large selection of different colored leaves and vegetables. Just add a little grated beet, snow peas, carrot, red bell peppers and some diced tomato or sun-dried tomatoes and you will have a rainbow of colored raw vegetables in one sitting.

Soup
Buy a pre-packaged selection of soup vegetables (discard the potato if there's one in the pack). Grate or dice the vegetables along with $6 - 8$ tomatoes (leave skin on tomatoes and other vegetables. Just scrub them well). Season your soups and vegetables dishes with natural spices e.g. Garlic, turmeric, cayenne pepper, cumin, oregano or Italian herbs and boil in plenty of filtered water. If you want to thicken the soup use Mung Dhal (check your health food shop).

Risotto

Place 2 cups of your homemade vegetable soup in a pot, and add 1 cup of cooked brown rice (your daily allowance). Stir over moderate heat until liquid has evaporated. Add a little more seasoning if desired.

Stir-fry

There is a wonderful selection of frozen stir-fry vegetable mixes in the freezer section of your local supermarket. Make sure you choose the one's with no added sauces.

There are also bags of prepared raw stir-fry vegetables in the fresh food section of your supermarket, though you will probably have to add more colors yourself.

Lentils

Buy a good selection of beans (black eyed, haricot, kidney, chickpeas etc) and cook about one fourth of them prior to starting the diet, or on the first day. These can be kept in the refrigerator and then added to salads and soups each day to create variety, and to act as 'tummy' fillers.

Doris's Salad (an example from someone who followed the diet)
Try this salad idea. ½ cup cooked chickpeas, ½ cup diced tomato, ½ diced avocado, a slice of onion diced finely, ½ cup diced mixed red and yellow capsicum, 1 tablespoon lemon juice.

In one serve, you have ½ a serve of lentils, ½ a piece of fruit and three colors of raw vegetables.

HELPFUL TIPS WHILST ON DANIEL'S DIET

- Drink 2 liters (2 quarts) of water daily. Mostly between meals but 1 glass during a meal is acceptable.
- Exercise should be minimal in the first 5 days, then if you're feeling well enough upgrade to moderate. After the 10 days keep upgrading consistently
- Ensure bowel regularity – see notes on natural laxatives.

- Taking a liver-cleansing supplement will help cleanse your system, especially for those with a history of alcohol or drug abuse, long-term clogged bowel, overeating issues and obesity.
- Eat breakfast and don't skip any meals.
- Eat 5 times per day. This is not a calorie restrictive diet, so don't go hungry. But don't overeat either, not even the good foods.

If you're craving sugar, add Stevia or ¼ tsp of unprocessed honey to your herbal tea, but only if necessary. It's good to train your taste buds to go without the sweet taste as this will help reprogram them to desire better food choices. Having said that, it's better to have a little honey and stay on the diet than not have it and stop the diet because of overwhelming sugar cravings. It's also better to have honey than any artificial sweetener.

Many people prefer warm meals, soups and steamed vegetables instead of salad, during the cold months; which is fine, but try to have as many raw salads as possible if you choose to undertake this diet in winter months.

Purchase all fruit and vegetables fresh as possible for better flavour. Eating ripe fruit is so much tastier and helps kids want more, if not ripe and poor quality then it can turn you off eating them. Cook vegetables so they are still crunchy – do not overcook.

Storage – keep all fruit and vegetables in the refrigerator crisper. Don't wash them until ready for use. Don't store in soft plastic or aluminium as they are toxic. Use hard plastic, cloth or paper.

CHAPTER FOURTEEN

YOUR 10 DAY EATING PLAN

I receive correspondence from readers of my books all over the world. North and South America, Australia, New Zealand, Africa, Great Britain, Europe, Asia, the Middle East, Singapore, Greece, Italy, Philippines etc. So I am well aware that people have different food choices, depending on where they live or their culture. The fantastic thing about Daniel's Way diet and why it is a **'Diet for Everybody'** is that it relies on food that is grown naturally and that means in whatever country or culture you live in. So simply use what is available to you. This book is truly a book suited to multiculturalism.

I am also well aware that people also appreciate a proven recipe format to follow, so as to make things easier and to make sure they are on the right program. However I encourage you to just follow the yes and no foods and create your own recipes and keep them simple and then you cannot go wrong – no matter where you live and even what budget you have.

Upon Rising
A large glass of water with a ½ lemon squeezed into it – or a teaspoon of organic apple cider vinegar. Drink 10- 20 minutes before eating. It aids digestion and is one of the best habits to get into, every day. (This is my start to the day)

Next:
45 minute brisk walk or bike ride; or whatever you enjoy most for exercise. I go for a 'prayer walk' every day, to pray and talk to God and ex-

ercise at the same time. I also take off my shoes and walk 20 minutes on grass or sand barefooted, this is a good general health tip - try it. Keep drinking more water to keep hydrated.

Followed by a dry skin brush before showering. Always use a natural bristled brush and don't be put off if it seems to sting the first few times you use it. It won't take long before you will enjoy it. This will help the elimination process for toxins being released through the skin.

PRE–BREAKFAST

Prunes in Squeezed Lemon Juice (10–20 minutes before breakfast)

Soak five or more prunes overnight in pure squeezed lemon juice. In the morning drink the juice and eat the prunes. This is good for everyone but especially those who may be constipated. If you need extra fibre, you can add psyllium husks.

Optional: Natural fiber; you can make a drink of psyllium husks in ½ glass of water, followed by another large glass of water. Use 1 tablespoon, depending on which brand. When you purchase it, ask what amounts to use and adjust it through practical experimentation to your individual system. Some people need more than others and when you visit the bathroom the result will tell you. If you are not noticing any bowel changes, you may need to increase the amount.

Do not underestimate the importance of prunes. Most people categorize them as just a laxative. Prunes do help your bowels but they are much more than that. They are a low-calorie fruit, packed with nutrients; high in potassium, iron, vitamin K, calcium and fibre and low in sodium. Adding them to your diet can help you attain better digestion and bowel action, better cardiovascular health, more energy and stronger bones.

Vegetable Juice
'How to preserve fresh vegetable juice'?

After juicing, fill to the top with your juice a glass container and seal. If the bottle is full the oxidation is slowed right down and you can safely have fresh juice for a good twelve hours without losing its nutritional value. If the container is 3/4 full or not sealed, oxidation takes place and the nutrients deteriorate rapidly.

Reminder: Drink two glasses per day and preferably 10 minutes or more before eating other meals. If you feel nauseas after drinking, this means it's too strong – don't be put off, dilute it down and sip slowly. You may need to have it with a meal, so it's mixed with other foods.

Note: Please allow an interval of 15 to 30 minutes after drinking vegetable juice and eating fruits. Some people may suffer from a slight stomach discomfort if they eat starchy food immediately after the vegetable juice or fruit.

BREAKFAST

It is essential that you eat breakfast. There are numerous studies which show that eating breakfast not only positively affects brain function, energy, and productivity for the rest of the day, but also contributes to weight loss. Basically breakfast kick-starts your metabolism. Breakfast is the time you sow nutrients into your body for energy for the first half of the day.

Even if you have never, or rarely, eaten breakfast, you can still train yourself to eat (and enjoy!) the most important meal of the day. It can simply be fruit for those who are in too much of a hurry or vegetable juice if you don't feel hungry – but it must be something. Change old thinking processes that suggest that by skipping meals you have to be better off in losing weight. It's just wrong information from past teaching or simply deception (lies) from the enemy (satan)'.

Something Hot

Don't be limited by traditional thinking about what you should have for breakfast. Especially in cold climates, you may need hot breakfasts. Why can't you have soup for breakfast? Heat up a left-over brown rice dish from the night before. One patient of mine who had just finished the Daniel's Diet told me she steamed vegetables for breakfast.

Do not eat breads on this diet. Most people eat too much bread; it will benefit you to have a break from it.

The idea is for you to be in control of your appetite and skipping meals may lead to you losing this control, making you feel so hungry you crave sugar/carbohydrates to give you instant gratification. It can also cause your metabolism to slow down to protect you from a perceived lack of food.

I do not recommend common packet cereals for breakfast. They are usually very high in sugar/salt (refined carbohydrate). If you eat common packet cereals regularly then you will eventually have energy slumps or fatigue.

In fact eating most commercial cereal for breakfast is no different to eating sweets for breakfast. Once the cereal reaches your stomach it is converted to sugar just like a plate of sweets. Would you eat Pudding for breakfast and pretend it Healthy?

Remember that a good wholesome breakfast (which includes a protein) and a light morning tea are really important for your blood sugar (energy) levels and hunger control. You don't need to eat a large amount, just learn to stop eating when you have had a sufficient amount.

MORNING & AFTERNOON TEA
Why Eating 5 times a Day is Beneficial
Eating something healthy between breakfast and lunch, and lunch and dinner, is recommended as it helps prevent hypoglycemia or the symptoms of low blood sugar and cravings for sugar and junk food. It will also boost your energy and concentration levels. The only times you should not eat between meals is if you are not having cravings and your energy and concentration are good.

Vegetable juice
If you haven't had vegetable juice earlier, then you can have it for morning tea.

Fruit; any choice – if you have not had it for breakfast – 3-4 pieces per day

Nuts & Seeds
Mixed or singular. (If you have allergy reaction to any nuts – don't have them).

The Biblical Energy Mix!
1 Samuel Chapter 30:12. *'And they gave him a piece of a cake of figs and two clusters of raisins. So when he had eaten, his strength came back to him; for he had eaten no bread nor drunk water for three days and three nights'.*

People with sugar-related problems during the 10-day diet may feel that they are getting weak, maybe getting the shakes or light headed. If so eat some pre-soaked dry fruit, just be sure not to eat too many. Soaking dried fruit (and nuts) in a small bowl of water rehydrates it, making it easily digestible.

Corn thins/Spelt cakes/Rice wafers
Check the labels – these convenient foods should be just corn and water or rice and water, therefore ok with this diet.

Spread with thinly sliced avocado with a sprinkle of cayenne pepper, Tamari soy sauce. If you do eat wafers, always add something nutritionally beneficial as they don't have much in themselves. Hummus and tomatoes are a good combination.

LUNCH
Create **Long-Lasting Energy**
One of the most common complaints I hear daily in my clinic is that people feel tired and lethargic after lunch. The main reason is that they are eating what I call 'heavy' non-essential food. It is heavy because it literally weighs you down to where you have little energy left. Foods like red meat, bread and most of the foods I mention in the 'NO' section of this book overload your body's digestive tract.

If you want to protect yourself from lethargy and energy drops, consider eating a light and easy-to-digest meal such as a salad. The benefits of this are enormous and far outweigh any 5 minute pleasure you get from refined carbohydrates and sweet, animal fatty, salty, (heavy) lunches.

Salads:

Salads are easy to take to work for lunch. They are also a fantastic accompaniment to your evening meal. Dress your salads with either fresh lemon or lime juice or lightly drizzle with extra virgin cold pressed olive oil, or flaxseed oil.

If using flaxseed oil, remember to store it in the fridge with the lid tightly closed as exposure to light and oxygen makes it go 'off' (rancid).

When making salads, let your imagination take off – use whatever vegetables you can think of. Try ones you have never heard of before. Check out the vegetable shops and think outside your normal choices – they are all created to enjoy. It is good for longevity of your healthy lifestyle to be able to create your own choices based on your favorite tastes.

If you are finding salad alone not filling, nor emotionally satisfying enough, add some soaked almonds or sliced avocado to expand your simple salad into a hearty meal.

Also, add nuts, seeds or lentils to your salad to make it more interesting and filling.

Alternatively, could also have a few tablespoons of mashed sweet potato or whole pieces of steamed sweet potato or brown rice, or rice as a 'side' with your salad.

Keep a container of grated carrot and grated beetroot (red beet) on-hand in the fridge. These are great additions to any salad or evening meal.

DINNER

If you eat a large meal at night, you are stocking up on energy (which remember, only comes from food) at the end of the day. You drop onto the couch and relax, which takes – NO energy. So what happens to all the excess from your main meal of the day? It goes straight to your thighs and stomach and eventually to your arteries and heart area. It's actually worse than that as it eventually causes intestinal problems and often insomnia and you then wake up the next morning feeling sluggish and awful. The beauty of Daniel's Diet is that all the foods should be 'light' on the tummy, but also keep this in mind for after the diet finishes.

The idea is to eat more during the day so you are not so hungry, and less at night. It helps to go for a walk after dinner to help settle the stomach or even do the housework – any moderate exercise will benefit you.

Brown rice and lentils can be added to dinner to make it more filling and help stop any excess cravings.

AFTER-DINNER SNACKS

Ok, we have all fallen into the trap of snacking after dinner. It's my own personal danger time, sitting there happily relaxed, (or lonely or bored) watching TV when my mind goes wandering to the fridge, chocolates or cookie jar.

If this sounds familiar, it is a good time to ask yourself some deep questions to judge your own habits: I will share this testimony with you:

One night I was bored watching TV and the phone rang, which ended up being an extreme emotionally stressful call. What was my reaction? I jumped up and started walking to the local deli with the intent to consume as much chocolate as I could lay my hands on. Half-way there I came to my senses and stopped, realizing that I really didn't need to be eating harmful food just to compensate for an emotional trigger.

I recognized my negative self-talk and that if I did carry on to the shop I would be giving in to the situation and would feel guilty and physically 'yuk' afterwards.

It was better to laugh at myself (which I did) and my reactions and change them to a positive. I did! I walked in the other direction and started praying and praising God and immediately I felt better and overcame not just the eating craving but it also made the emotional situation easier to handle. Try it – next time your 'buttons' are pushed, dare to react differently (resist the enemy and he will have to flee from you.) If you do this enough times you set up a positive habit or reaction to stress, boredom etc. then you have the victory.

Practical Advice

It is best not to eat in the evening but if you have to eat something, make it healthy (low GI) and light on the stomach. Perhaps celery/carrot sticks and hummus dip or a piece of low GI fruit (remember you don't want to be eating high GI foods before bed – the energy has no time to burn up and fat gain results.) A handful of nuts and seeds should help.

CHAPTER FIFTEEN

SETTING GOALS IS THE FIRST STEP TO SUCCESS

Set Your Personal Goals

Setting goals is the first step to success.

Goals provide you with the focus needed to achieve what you desire, and creates the motivation and will power to fulfill the goals that you set.

In fact, the single most important factor in a diet or weight loss program is having committed goals. Studies indicate that people who write down their goals succeed in achieving them over 50 percent more than those who don't write down goals.

Personal Goals for the next 10 Days

Name:..

Commence Date:........................ **Finish Date:**.............................

Weight: Now:........................ **Finish:**......................................

MEASUREMENTS	
	WAIST Now:........................ Finish:......................
CHEST Now........................ Finish:......................	
	THIGHS Now:................... Finish:...............
HIPS Now:..................... Finish:..................	UPPER ARMS Now:................... Finish:................

Current health symptoms before starting:

_____

_____

What's Most Important? List your three most important goals:

_____

_____

_____

What could get in My Way? List some obstacles to accomplishing your goals:

_____

_____

_____

My Personal Affirmations are:

_____

_____

_____

_____

My Pledge

"I will commit to the Daniel's Way health plan and acknowledge that I may not always stick to the plan and when that happens I won't beat myself up, rather I will get back on track with the next meal."
"I will give it 100% effort and stick to 10 days"

Print Name:_____

Sign Name: _____

To commit to a healthier lifestyle

What Are the Benefits for You?

Understanding the benefits you can achieve in this 10 day program can be a great motivator to follow the plan and achieve your goals..

The benefits are outstanding:

There are many testimonies to prove this diet will benefit you. The following are to encourage you and show you why you need to have a healthy lifestyle, and some practical ways to enjoy the diet.

It's going To Help You:

- Lose weight
- Get more energy (overcome tiredness)
- Detoxify your body
- Clear your mind & sharpen your concentration
- Restore a good acid/alkaline balance to your body
- Stimulate the proper functions of organs and tissue
- Stabilize your emotions
- Recognize and overcome food allergies & addictions
- Overcome hypoglycaemia (sugar problems) and Insulin resistance
- Improve your skin and hair texture
- Regain & maintain your health
- Help prevent cancer and other diseases
- Help recover from illness and drug treatments
- Enhance you spiritually

There is more;

- It can save your life
- It makes your life of better quality – you enjoy life more
- You look and feel better
- Less sickness and disease
- It can improve your sex life
- More confidence & improved self image
- Improved concentration
- More productive –you can achieve more
- You can fit into your favourite clothes again
- You can gain control back in your life.

Help to Stay on Track:

Planning your meals in advance and sticking to this plan will keep you accountable of the foods you eat and will help you to stick to your program.

Stick to a shopping list to avoid impulse purchases and purchasing foods that are not on the allowable food list. Always do your food shopping on a full stomach. It is easier to make the right choices when you are not hungry.

Remove as much food as practical from your home that is not on the allowable food list. Remember: "If it's in front of you it will eventually be eaten".

Ensure you have a good support network. Tell your friends and family that you are on the program, your reasons and motivations for doing it and how important your goals are to you. Try and get an exercise 'buddy'. Ask them to be supportive and not offer you junk foods etc. as it only makes it harder for you.

There is a support at my website *www.wisdomforhealth.com*

If making meals in advance split into correct serving sizes and refrigerate or freeze immediately

Drinking a large glass of water before your meal will make you feel full and help to avoid over eating.

Learn to say "no" to temptation and "stop" when feeling full. Remember eat slowly and at the table and not in front of TV is wise. Try not to have sweets and cookies in the house. Remove the temptation.

The next step is to get God's help by laying a scriptural foundation for the 10 days on the diet.

CHAPTER SIXTEEN

SCRIPTURE SUPPORT

Your 10 Days Scripture declarations

'I will agree with you (in prayer) for success on this diet and for your health and healing.' (Philip)

Matthew 18:19. *"Again I say to you that if two of you agree on earth concerning anything that they ask, it will be done for them by My Father in heaven."*

Day One

Your Scripture for the day:

"But Daniel made up his mind that he would not defile himself with the King's choice of food or with wine ..." (Daniel 1:8 NASB)

"...their fruit will be for food and their leaves for medicine." (Ezekiel 46:22)

Make up your mind what you really want to achieve from going on this diet. Write down these goals then resolve in your heart and mind to complete the ten days. It's vital that you mentally prepare and desire to do the diet and that you anticipate the rewards you'll obtain by finishing it.

Be determined to overcome the doubts, fears and former negative thinking that your mind may throw up to stop you getting to where you want to be.

Overcoming mind battles is the biggest key to success. Note that even Daniel, to complete the ten days, had to set his mind to resist peer pressure, hunger pangs, temptation of foods and doubts. If you become determined in your mind and heart then succeeding becomes a probability not a possibility.

It more than simply wanting to do it; it has to be a strong desire based on the knowledge you have now gained from reading this book. **Knowledge followed by action will bring success.**

Day Two

Your Scripture for the day:

"I can do all things through Christ, who strengthens me." (Philippians 4:13 KJV)

The first 3 days are usually the hardest. If you are suffering headaches or nausea, feeling weak or hungry – then say and believe this Scripture as a positive affirmation. The headaches and any other withdrawal symptoms are a sign that the diet is working, they should pass within three or four days. If they don't – stop the diet and seek a naturopath's advice to find out why. Make sure you are eating five times a day and, if possible, try not to take painkillers.

You can do it! Maybe now is the time to think about what healthy gift you will give yourself when you successfully reach Day 11.

Day Three

Your Scripture for the day:

"And they gave him a piece of a cake of figs and two clusters of raisins. So when he had eaten, his strength came back to him; for he had eaten no bread nor drunk water for three days and three nights." (1 Samuel 30:12)

If you are feeling weak and craving sugar make sure that between meals you are eating the energy mix recommended on this diet (almonds, pumpkin and sunflower seeds etc), sun dried fruits may be included for the sugar craving. Drink 2 quarts of water, with some squeezed lemon juice added occasionally.

Day Four

Your Scripture for the day:

"Therefore do not cast away your confidence, which has great reward. For you have need of endurance, so that after you have done the will of God, you may receive the promise." (Hebrews 10:35-36)

Often on fasts your feelings (senses) are heightened and it is not uncommon for people to be emotionally sensitive. Some people report that they weep easily at different stages of the fast. This is normal under the circumstances and if you understand what is happening it isn't a problem. Actually it's the opposite; you can learn a lot about yourself at these times. It's very beneficial to write everything down so later when you are not so fragile you can sort them out in an appropriate manner. One of the blessings of fasting is to become more spiritually sensitive (alert), more 'aware' and hear from God. By writing things down you don't forget and then afterwards you can ascertain if it was just emotional or was it really God guiding you. If it warrants further insight or explanation, seek wise council from a trusted person (pastor) or group.

If doubts and fears are coming into your mind, remember your reasons for doing this diet. Re-read the sections of this book that are relevant to your situation. The Bible says don't lose confidence because if you don't it will bring a great reward.

Day Five

Your Scripture for the day:

"I say then: walk in the Spirit, and you shall not fulfill the lusts of the flesh. For the flesh lusts against the Spirit, and the Spirit against the flesh; and these are contrary to one another, so that you do not do the things that you wish." (Galatians 5:16 – 17)

By now your body is enjoying the healing process that is taking place internally. Going off harmful foods and fasting is akin to giving your stomach and intestines a holiday. So be encouraged to keep eating only the good, healthy food, remembering they are the ones that contain life and healing properties. Let your spiritual side take charge over your physical and soul sides. Make this diet a spiritual experience and a time for you to take back control.

Day Six

Your Scripture for the day:

But His (Jesus) answer was: "My grace is all you need, for My power is greatest when you are weak". I am most happy, then, to be proud of my weakness, in order to feel the protection of Christ's power over me." (2 Corinthians 12:9 GNB)

You are past the half way mark now, beneficial things are happening, whether you are aware of them or not. Take this opportunity to trust God to see you through any healing situation – whether physical, emotional or spiritual. Many people have testified that prayer not only made this diet easier but also made it a profoundly positive experience, so don't hesitate to pray and rely on God for help. If you're feeling like you can't keep going remember God's Grace is sufficient for you.

Day Seven

Your Scripture for the day:

God… "Who pardons all your iniquities; Who heals all your diseases." (Psalm 103:2)

Have faith that healing and weight loss are taking place inside you, more and more every day. No matter how big or small a problem you now have, through Jesus all healing is possible. Keep praying and believing.

You are doing your part to enhance healing to your mind, body and emotions, ask and trust God to do the rest. Remember this diet is based on His Word, The Bible.

Day Eight

Your Scripture for the day:

"Beloved, I pray that you may prosper in all things and be in good health, just as your soul prospers." (3 John 1:2)

Pat yourself on the back, its day eight already. Remember the benefits; it's worth it.

Being in good health all the time is possible, if you learn to change and follow a healthy lifestyle. This diet gives you the key to detoxification and launching into a healthy future. I too pray that you prosper in all things - body, soul and spirit because without health in each of these three areas you cannot enjoy life to its fullest.

Day Nine

Your Scripture for the day:

"If you forgive others the wrongs they have done to you, your Father in heaven will also forgive you. But if you do not forgive others, then your Father will not forgive the wrongs you have done." (Matthew 6:14-15 TEV)

Take the opportunity to realize that you have completed nine days of a partial fast. Any addictions or emotional hurts from the past can now be let go. Any bitterness or unforgiveness you may retain can be released and when it is, you too are released from its ramifications. Set yourself free from any negative issues you harbor because otherwise they will eventually cause ill health and co-dependencies. It is up to you.

True health comes from physical, emotional and spiritual fulfillment. Every feeling we experience is faithfully recorded in every living cell. Indeed your individual feelings have a specific effect on certain cells or body areas. Fear, anger, resentment and all negative emotions take their toll physically, spiritually as well as emotionally. Loving thoughts, positive words and appropriate actions not only strengthen us but also allow our body to fight back against the effects of disease.

Unforgiveness is a huge hindrance to your spiritual health. On the other hand, forgiveness, joy and laughter have awesome healing power.

"Being cheerful keeps you healthy. It is slow death to be gloomy all the time." (Proverbs 17:22. TEV)

This was quoted many thousands of years ago and science today tells us laughter and joy release certain endorphins in our brain that make us feel great. Happiness, positivity and laughter have a very positive impact on our health.

Day Ten

Your Scripture for the day:

"… Oh that you would bless me indeed, and enlarge my territory, and that your hand would be with me, and that you would keep me from evil. That I may not cause pain. So God granted him what he requested." (1 Chronicles 4:10)

You have reached the last day. Now is the time to start planning for the future. If you want to go on with the diet for another 5-10 or 20 days don't stop. Use wisdom and monitor how you are feeling and press on. Remember you can undertake the diet as often as you desire.

If you have been praying specifically for something, then as this scripture states, believe this –"So God granted him (you) what (you) he requested."

Day Eleven - the day after

"Afterwards Jesus found him in the temple, and said to him, "See, you have been made well. Sin no more, lest a worse thing come upon you." (John 5:14 NKJV)

The scripture quote for today really says it all. The biggest reason for people not maintaining their goal weight after a special diet is because they fall back into old habits and routines. Don't go back to the same old lifestyle as you had pre -diet.

Congratulations!

Give yourself a pat on the back and say, **"Well done, I deserve a reward."**

Give yourself a treat; obviously not a food based treat that will undo all your good efforts but treat yourself to something else that you enjoy. Buy yourself something special, have a massage, go out for the evening to a show, get a new hair style ….

Many will have lost weight; have increased energy and mental clarity, a decrease in body aches and pains, improved vision and improved texture of your skin. Others may have accomplished spiritual goals. It's always good to write down anything accomplished and give thanks to God.

Please email to my clinic and give your testimony to encourage others, I will post it on my website (no real names used). Also send in any recipe tips that you found helpful.

My address is found at the back of this book.

PART FOUR

POST DIET

CHAPTER SEVENTEEN

KEEP THE MOMENTUM

"What now?" you may well ask.

First compare the records of how you were before and after the 10-day detox program.

Congratulate yourself on the changes, no matter how large or small they may be. Appreciate the changes you have been able to create in such a short time.

It's very important when coming off a partial fast to not go overboard with your eating. Your stomach has been eating healthy foods for ten days, and it's starting to shrink. It is not wise to overload it now with previously banned foods.

If you go out and have a big feast e.g. fast foods, hamburger and fries it will be bad for your whole system. You will immediately be putting toxins, sugar and saturated fat back into your body and overloading your digestion. By now you should know what they are doing to your body. As a rule of thumb, the same amount of time should be given to the post diet as spent on the program. Your first meals should continue to be small amounts regularly. Then each day introduce a food that you desire. Foods to include are fish and some whole grains into your diet. Next, include free range eggs (soft boiled, omelets or poached), a good wholesome rye or wholegrain bread. If you have any bad reactions to any food, its clearly a warning and not for you.

Then after 5-7 days slowly introduce red meat if you so choose.

Try and stay away from all the foods you now know are traps, use all the information you have learnt to set up your eating habits from now on. Your body needs at least two months of a constant new weight to lock in a new set-point weight. Once you reach that level it's easier to maintain your desired weight. This gives you a time goal of two months from now, to work at your diet and lifestyle. Get to that time or level and you will find it's not that difficult to maintain your weight and health.

Today is a critical time in this diet. Your decision now will determine your future health and weight maintenance. Consider it carefully.

What to do next?

Congratulations on completing the 10 day diet.

My goals are to give every one, step by step instruction and answers to your individual situation. So that in a few short weeks you will have reached your goals of losing weight and having more energy and feeling very healthy. The end result being that you get into the 'zone' of living a lifestyle that ensures you don't go back to where you used to be, but maintain your good weight and health. So this healthy lifestyle becomes the new normal for you, and you automatically choose to eat and shop the right way for you. Then you are truly 'free'.

The next step is to keep the momentum going to reach your goals and I offer the following to help you achieve just that.

If you have not lost enough weight and want to lose more I suggest my next step diet and weight loss plan. **'The 6 Week Low Carb Diet'**. This book can only be purchased from my web site. www.wisdomforhealth.com

This plan is nearly the opposite of this 10 day vegetarian diet. The effect of doing these two diets in tandem is very powerful and has wonderful results. You should lose 2 Kg a week and continue your journey to success. This diet plan is not long term and 6 weeks should be enough and then you can revisit Daniel's Diet again. Keep in mind you can reintroduce this 10 day plan at any time and as often as you want. You may continue for longer than the 10 days if you are feeling good.

Long Term Diet Plan

Moderation - What Is It?

In my observations, people pay lip service to the word 'moderation'. They may say it and even think it, but in reality don't really know what it means. My definition of moderation is, eat 75% natural foods and 25% other, the 75 – 25 plan. This rule of thumb means on your plate you have 75% salad or vegetables and the 25% is meat, pasta or whatever you want. Not the other way around. You should also eat slowly, stopping before you feel completely full as it takes time for your mind to recognize that you are actually full. This will prevent overeating and therefore is part of the moderation principle.

Now is Your Chance to Overcome Old Harmful Eating Habits.

By now after reading this book it should be clear that changing old thought patterns and eating habits is essential not only for weight loss but for ongoing good health. To encourage you even further let me show you typical eating habits of the average person.

The Typical Western Daily Diet:

Breakfast: Packet Cereal, oat porridge with milk and sugar, toast with jam/jello, coffee/tea, orange juice – or skip breakfast and eat nothing.

Morning tea: Muffin, biscuit or cake, coffee (includes packet iced coffee). High carb - 'health bar'.

Lunch: Sandwich, meat pie, 'take out" or bread roll and a soft drink/ soda, fruit juice or caffeine drink. Hot French fries (chips), white rice, packet noodles….

Afternoon tea: Sweetened Yoghurt, Crackers/cheese, sweet biscuits, chocolate and more caffeine.

Dinner: Pasta, white rice, 2-3 veggie e.g. potato/peas/kale, bread, meat followed by sweets or cheese and savory biscuit and alcohol.

TV snacks: Chocolate, ice cream, packet chips/crisps, candy (lollies), salted peanuts etc

This eating lifestyle is disastrous. You have put yourself on a 24-hour continuous cycle of craving more and more carbohydrates or sug-

ar. This can lead to cravings you won't be able to control.
Why?

This habitual way of eating is over stimulating your appetite-control mechanism.

By eating too many sugars, stimulants and refined carbs daily you activate an addiction for more of the same type of foods. This addiction makes you want or crave more and more of the very food you know is causing your weight gain. In other words the more sugar and refined carbs you eat the more you desire to eat them. To win over weight gain you must break this cycle of craving and you can. The less you consume them the less power the addiction has on you and you then can say no to eating them. The Bible says *'Resist the enemy and he has to flee from you''*, (James 4.7) well if you resist harmful cravings often enough the cravings will disappear from you also. After about twenty one days your taste buds don't need the taste of sugar, chocolate or iced coffee as much and eventually you can eat small amount without falling into the addictive cycle again. But first you must gain control of the cravings.

When I was a young I used to have two heaped teaspoons of sugar in my daily six to eight cups tea and coffee. Each day I'd eat half a packet of cookies plus, ice cream or chocolate, white bread, packet cereal with another tablespoon of sugar, and consume alcohol. I changed – so can you. I enjoy my food much more now than then and if just a pinch of instant sugar was added to my cup of tea, I wouldn't be able to drink it. It tastes revolting.

Are you addicted?

Try going completely without your most commonly eaten sugar, refined carbohydrate food and caffeine for 3 -4 days. After this time, you should be in no doubt, one way or another, as to whether you are addicted. The symptoms will not lie; craving, withdrawals, headaches, irritability, etc, will manifest if you are addicted.

The teaching in this book will break you out of this cycle and set you free from cravings. The only way to do this is to change your lifestyle. And if you can do that, being enslaved by cravings and frustrated by long-term weight gain will no longer be a problem.

I believe– 'Diet-related chronic diseases as the single largest cause of death in Western society'. This book teaches you to recognize and choose to avoid some of the modern foods and eat more of Gods created foods and if you do you will experience better health and overcome weight problems.

Let's do something about it, it's never too late, you do not have to be a statistic.

What to Eat After the 10 Days

You have completed the 10 days or more – the question is what do I do next?

You are now at the crossroad of decision for your future. You have 4 choices.

1. Do you choose to continue on as a vegetarian?

2. Do you choose to live a life based on the moderation principle?

3. Do you choose to succumb and turn back to your old habits?

4. Do you choose to go on my 'low carb diet' to lose more weight?

Wisdom says; don't go back to your old ways, as this is how you got overweight or toxic in the first place. Any percentage of change from where you were before doing this diet is a plus for your future long term health. For example; if you give up one of your most dangerous foods and cut down on two others, this is good, don't underestimate what you have achieved by this change. You don't have to eat perfectly, so don't put that pressure on yourself, it's a recipe for failure. If you change just 30% from pre diet then you can expect a 30% improvement in your long term health.

Base Your Future Lifestyle around Gods Way of eating

You can choose to stay on this principle of vegetarian eating or choose to include meat and other food choices back into your diet. You simply add (include) different healthy foods to what you have just learnt to do with this diet plan.

Whatever you do, progress continually towards following Gods principles for health.

Although the scriptures don't say how long Daniel followed this vegetarian diet, it is indicated he continued in this way for at least the three years he was at the training centre (Daniel 1:12- 16). However his people were not normally vegetarian.

Philip's Guide to continued health and healing

I suggest you read my book series to gain knowledge and wisdom for a long term lifestyle of health, happiness and enjoying foods. You are free to eat whatever you want, your body is your responsibility and I know that now you have read this book you will choose well.

PART FIVE

FREQUENTLY ASKED QUESTIONS

CHAPTER EIGHTEEN

FAQ

Q. 'I have an Allergy to Wheat and Gluten – is this diet suitable for me?'

Yes this is a Gluten and wheat free diet.
In my clinic I have lost count of the amount of people that have had reversals of health problems when I put them on a wheat free diet. A large part of the immense success of this diet plan is that it has NO wheat, sugar, alcohol, dairy or caffeine in it. You do need whole grains in your every day diet, however look outside the normal and use other grains. Brown rice is one great option.

Hidden gluten can be found in soy sauce and is why I recommend the Tamari – wheat free soy sauce. If you have severe gluten intolerance - it is crucial to read labels prior to purchasing food products.

REMEMBER: Always check the labels on the foods you eat – you'll be surprised what seemingly 'harmless' foods actually contain.

There are Delicious Alternatives to Wheat!
1. Coconut flour
2. Buckwheat flour is gluten free
3. Millett
4. Quinoa
5. Corn

Take millet as an example; you can eat it for breakfast, use millet sprouts in salads or as flour for baking. It has about 15% protein content, contains B vitamins, minerals (including magnesium and iron), vitamin E and phytic acid. It may help in lowering cholesterol (contains niacin). It has good fiber content and if stored in airtight containers, in cool conditions it keeps fresh for months.

Gluten is a high allergenic food and most people would benefit from either eliminating it or severely reducing it from their diet. Often, if you remove allergenic foods (e.g. Dairy and grains/bread/pasta etc) from your diet, your cravings for sweets will get less and less. Even your mood will improve, your weight will drop, and your overall health will improve.

Reminder; Rye, spelt, barley, oats and couscous contain gluten.

Q. "Can I Take a Protein Powder on This Diet"?

Yes you can.

At first thought it might seem to be getting away from the original idea of a Biblical diet however, by using a protein powder it's really only utilizing modern technology to make things easier for some people to complete the diet. After all, it's only food crushed into a powder.

It's an option I would encourage for:

- Underweight and debilitated people
- For those who crave sugar or food so much that they can't stay on the diet for long as they keep giving in to their cravings
- For those people who are simply too busy to prepare and eat correctly on the diet.
- For anyone who is run down and over stressed.
- For those who want to continue the diet past the ten days.
- If the protein powder is going to be the difference between you completing this diet and not, then use it.

Suggestions

There are many products available that should not be used on this diet (or anytime). They will be counterproductive to what we are trying to achieve. If in doubt don't use any.

The reason I say this is three fold; firstly some of these protein or weight loss products contain too much sugar or carbohydrate and not enough protein. Have a close look at the nutritional panel and compare the carbohydrate (sugar) count to the protein. Many manufacturers replace fat content with sugar and promote the low fat aspect. As we have already discussed, excess sugar is toxic and over stimulates insulin, a hormone that then converts and stores this sugar as body fat. I am not saying you cut out all carbohydrates in your diet, but for sustained weight loss, you will need to balance your intake of unrefined carbohydrates with adequate protein and the right protein powder can be very helpful in achieving this balance. This balance will reduce insulin secretions to appropriate levels so you can utilize incoming food for energy and not store it as body fat. The use of any sugar on this diet is not recommended. Secondly; the use of artificial sweeteners is counterproductive to a detox program, unless it is herbal like stevia. Thirdly; the protein base must consist of a low allergenic natural food base.

The good news is that the right type of protein shakes are wonderful help for weight management because they boost metabolism, naturally suppress appetite and offset the weight gaining effects of insulin. To aid people to continue past the ten days, keep their cravings under control and to help continue the stimulation of weight loss, then you can add a protein shake.

So, which are the right ones? The sugar (carbohydrate) content must be much lower than the protein content (the lower the better) and it must also be low in fat. It should contain no artificial sweeteners, flavors or colors. On this Diet you can use Rice Protein Concentrate (non- GMO), or Pea Protein Isolate as it is vegetarian based (dairy free). The formulas made from whey isolate or concentrate can be good quality, but because the source is from Dairy (animal) they shouldn't be used on the detox diet, after is ok if you haven't got severe lactose intolerance. Definitely no soy based shakes as soy may be counterproductive to some people.

Q. "I have been prayed for at my church and am believing God for my healing. Is it a lack of faith and trust in God's

Supernatural healing to do this diet, and take herbs and vitamins?"

No it's not. In fact, by following this diet you are putting faith into action, which always brings a result. It's a step of obedience to take an active role in looking after 'The temple of the Holy Spirit' (your body), and obedience always brings a reward and in this situation expect a healing reward. As for taking herbs and vitamins, God created them in our food, for our benefit and use, therefore its wisdom and maturity to take them when needed, or as a preventative measure. They are, after all, God's medicinal gift to us.

I see it as working with Jesus for your healing and not against Him. If you do your part, then God will do His. For example, if you have high cholesterol, high blood pressure, or are overweight, it's highly likely to have been caused in the first place by your eating habits and lifestyle. In other words, you are causing the symptoms by what you are doing or not doing. Therefore, common sense should tell you to change what's causing the problem in the first place. Yes, God does heal supernaturally, but He is God not your personal genie and you must be careful not to be presumptuous in your thinking.

It's important to understand God's health and healing principles.

There are three types of healing
  (1) The supernatural miracles,
  (2) The natural i.e. herbal medicine, diet, fasting, medicine etc
  (3) The genetic process of healing (our immune system).

When you blend the natural and the spiritual together you have an awesome combination, do it now and see what God will do.

It should increase your faith and potential to be healed if you commit to Jesus, "I'm willing to follow your health principles, Lord, and change my bad habits. I believe I will be healed and set free of all physical and emotional problems in the Name of Jesus." Following Daniel's Diet together with meditating on healing scriptures, you are now putting your faith into action and positioning yourself to receive healing from Jesus.

If you are supernaturally healed, great, but if you don't want the sickness to come back at a later date you must change your lifestyle. You can't keep expecting God to heal you, without you doing or changing anything. God is probably waiting for you to do this diet and take His herbs and vitamins. He is waiting for you to do your part and then He will do His.

God heals through herbal medicine:
In Isaiah Ch. 38.1 we are told Hezekiah was sick and near death through a boil that was infecting him, and God told him he was going to die. Hezekiah cried out to God to be healed. In response, God healed him and added fifteen years to his life. But look at how God healed him! 'Now Isaiah had said, *"Let them take a lump of figs, and apply it as a poultice on the boil, and he shall recover."'* (v.21). I find it fascinating that God healed Hezekiah through an herbal treatment. Obviously God did not build a wall between faith, miracles and using natural (herbal) medicine.

In summary:
We are free from Old Testament or Mosaic laws that put restrictions on certain foods. However, with this freedom of choice comes more responsibility - the responsibility to choose wisely and follow God's Health Principles. It does not give us permission to go open slather and eat anything and everything. Don't get me wrong, food is to be enjoyed, but everything in moderation. So whilst we are no longer under law we do have the responsibility of choosing to be obedient to God's Health principles.

When you add prayer and faith in Jesus to following a healthy lifestyle, you have the most potent healing force available to us.

Having knowledge of God's principles for health enables us to travel the daily walk of faith. And with more power through our understanding and application of God's instruction in our daily lives, i.e. faith and obedience, this becomes a powerful way to stand in faith and resist the enemy in our physical health.

This book offers a balance between physical obedience and divine healing.

Q. "Will Daniel's Diet Help My Health Problems?"

Yes it can. The philosophy behind these lifestyle changes is to free the body of blockages so it can respond properly and create the right environment so that it heals itself. Many positive results will happen if you give your body the chance to right itself. The Daniel's Diet does not cure or treat any disease specifically. Its primary role is to be a catalyst for the body's powerful regenerating and rebuilding capabilities through detoxification. Improving the body's natural immune function and experiencing weight loss are (simply put), a few of the wonderful side effects of Daniel's Diet.

Daniel's Diet is the first step in getting you on the road to change so that many symptoms of ill health are diminished. Adding supplements enhances your body's ability to fix itself.

One of the wonderful things about this diet is that after you finish it – what happens or does not happen will tell a lot about your personal health status and metabolism. From this knowledge you can then work an individualized diet and health plan to reach your goals of weight loss and abundant health.

Q. "I'm Iron deficient and currently taking iron tablets and I eat meat daily to improve my Iron intake. Can I do this diet?"

Yes you can. However, if you are extremely weak physically then my advice is to first check with your doctor. For those who are in the general anemic category, go ahead and do this diet, make sure you are eating lots of leafy green vegetables, checking the food lists previously mentioned so that you can include plenty of Iron rich foods in your meals.

Make sure you take an Iron supplement as well. I prefer a natural (herbal) Iron liquid tonic because it is very easily absorbed and prevents digestion problems and constipation. If any iron supplement causes any stomach issues – stop it and go onto a more natural formula. There are also natural Iron capsules which are good. The better quality ones will include in the mix added Vitamin B12, C, and Folic acid. This combination will help absorption and prevents the stomach problems often associated with Iron medication.

Q. "What If I Don't Lose Weight?"

There is always a reason if you can't lose weight. You just have to find it. Doing this diet is not a waste of your time even if you don't lose much weight initially. It will still help detoxify your system and make you aware of the underlying reason working against your success. Often the reason is physical, but sometimes it can also be emotional or spiritual.

Finding the core of the problem is part of the aim of this book. If you pursue your individual issue then healing and weight loss will eventuate. Whatever you do, don't just accept your situation. If you desire to get well and do something about your weight, you will get results.

I have had people consult with me after seeing multiple practitioners and researching many avenues themselves. Invariably they find the answer to their individual problem, if they keep seeking the answers. I believe God will direct your footsteps if you are willing, and reading this book may well be the answer to your prayers, but even so you still have to do your part. You can't pray the calories or sugar out of your triple sized hamburger, soda and fries – we wish!. I often have patients specifically fly across the continent or drive over 10 hours for a consultation. Yet others complain if they have to cross the metro area. Priorities, determination and commitment will get you powerful results. I often say that 'if' you follow my instructions and work with me, eventually you will get your desired result. It is the 'if' part that seems the hardest issue.

(I discuss all the reasons for stubborn weight loss in detail in my second book – Daniel's Diet Lifestyle).

Case History

A very overweight lady completed Daniel's Diet and after ten days she said she felt a lot better in herself but had not lost any weight. She decided to do another ten days because she was feeling good but she still lost only a very small amount.

I suggested she consult with me privately so that we could find the reasons why she wasn't experiencing weight loss. The result showed she had multiple long-standing health issues. I decided a Hair Tissue Analysis was needed and requested she check her *Resting Basal Body Temperature for four mornings in succession to check for sluggish metabolism (thyroid). From this simple test we discovered she had an under active thyroid. She also needed hormone and liver support. Now we were getting to the root cause of her problem (thyroid, liver, hormones and self-image). The hair analysis showed that she had mineral imbalances and had excess copper and lead in her system, which we needed to rectify.

Treatment with herbs and minerals commenced and she slowly started to lose weight from then on. We were still using Daniel's Diet as the foundation of her treatment but adding some additional healthy protein to the diet. The self-image improved with some counseling, and her success at losing weight helped here also.

Refer to chapter 5 for more details on how to do the Basal Body Temperature Test.

Q. "What herbs and spices can you use to flavor your vegetables?"

Add garlic, turmeric, cayenne pepper, ginger, mixed herbs, natural curry powder, basil, bay leaves, rosemary, thyme, chili peppers – anything grown naturally and has nothing else added to it is acceptable. All herbs and spices are good but the key to using them is they must be in their most natural state. No processed foods or foods soaked in vinegar, sugar or salt can be used, (you can't wash tinned beets for example; you must use fresh grown ones). Check all labels.

Q. "What if my bowels slow down?"
Sometimes a change of diet can affect your bowel movements. This reaction is common, however it is not good for what you are trying to achieve. It is very important to keep your bowels regular, so if they become sluggish, take some Psyllium husks and/or drink prune juice, eat prunes and dried figs.

If this doesn't work – then a natural laxative is ok to use in the short term.

*Re-read the section on constipation in this book and this should fix the problem, if problems persist, please consult a naturopath or doctor.

Q. "Can I do Daniel's Diet if I am Pregnant?"
NO - I would not advise any pregnant woman to do the diet unless under medical supervision. Although beneficial to the mother, it's not clear about the effects of toxins being released on the fetus. Daniel's Diet per se may not be advisable but certainly a healthy modified diet would be. In other words, eat a diet based on vegetables, fruit and seeds, with the addition of fish, eggs, complex carbohydrates and lean meat, but always be under a doctor's advice just to be sure.

Q. I Have a History of Infertility, will Daniel's diet help me to conceive a baby?"
This is an interesting question and the answer is yes - it is possible. It has been my experience that some female patients who have not been able to fall pregnant, have conceived after completing Daniel's Diet, and using specific herbs. It is a well-known fact that chemical toxins can block conception. It would be beneficial for all pre conception to do this diet. What happens is that the diet and change in lifestyle enables the body to detoxify itself? This in turn improves the natural flow of the body's hormones. Furthermore, by using specific nutrients and herbs to stimulate different physiological actions (that may have been imbalanced) the body begins to rectify itself, allowing conception. In fact, I am currently consulting with a patient, who has just had a baby girl; she had been try-

ing for many years to get pregnant. She changed her lifestyle, completed Daniel's Diet and with the addition of an herbal supplement became pregnant less than three months after ending the diet!

Q. "What if, during the 10 days, I make a mistake and eat something wrong or get depressed, have a bad night and binge?"

My answer is don't feel guilty, there is no reason to beat yourself up (no condemnation). I personally have started the diet and for whatever reason stopped on day 3,4 or 5 many times.

If you are having a bad emotional attack or are really feeling depressed, then stop the diet. Do what you can under your circumstance, but keep making changes, keep a forward momentum going, even if its one food at a time. Eventually you will achieve your breakthrough.

If you just have one bad day, simply, start up again from the next meal or the next day. It is like going on a trip in your car and getting a flat tire. You don't turn back because of the flat tire you just change it and keep going. The worst thing you could do is give up. You can still get the results if you keep going!

Q. "What if i am a Cigarette Smoker?"

Ideally you should give up smoking before you start the diet, but I know that many won't be able to. My advice is to still do the diet and aim for this partial fast to be the catalyst for you to give it up. I have seen many people with food addictions overcome them by fasting, so I believe the same is possible for smokers. If you are smoking, it will hinder rather than help with detoxing, but the diet will still be very beneficial for you in other areas. So, do it anyway!

Q. "What if I am Struggling with Anorexia or Bulimia?"

If you have tendencies towards either of these two problems you must do the diet under supervision. The diet will not cause people to become anorexic or bulimic and in a lot of cases it may even be a big help in getting someone who is anorexic/bulimic back into normal eating patterns.

One anorexic patient I treated was barely eating anything at all. I encouraged her by explaining to her that vegetable juices would not cause her to put on any weight. This took a while but she eventually trusted me enough to start drinking juices and taking some vitamin and mineral supplements.

Once some good nutrition got into her system she became more rational in her thinking, so eventually started eating fruit. Over time this progressed to the Daniel's Diet and then to a normal vegetarian lifestyle. The result was that she overcame the anorexia and led a normal life from then on. She has two children now which is fantastic because when she was anorexic her menstruation stopped and the chances of becoming pregnant were nigh impossible.

One of the hardest things dealing with chronic anorexics I have found is their mental state. It can be very frustrating trying to 'get through' to them, the advice you give just doesn't seem to register properly. One important reason is that they are not getting enough nutrition to allow their brains biochemistry to function properly. This is why they must be treated holistically.

I am currently treating a bulimic patient who is progressing very well; she is currently eating 2 meals per day without vomiting (previously vomiting after every meal). I am using the same protocol as with the anorexic patient. This person is a leader in her Church and has a wonderful home environment, however no one knows about her problem. She is fearful of church people critically judging her and too worried even to see the counselors in case they 'talk', so she hides it. Because patients feel and are safe talking with me they 'open up' and this in itself is very beneficial and part of the healing process.

It is very important to have a non-judgmental, understanding of their predicament and to offer them not only spiritual help, but also an emotional and a physical plan. A plan they can accept and therefore desire to work within their situation. Not rushing, or pushing them, but understanding and working closely with them, in love and compassion. It will help bring a positive change in their mind and healing normality results.

Q. "What do i do if i go out to café or restaurant while on this diet?"

Instead of meeting friends for coffee/lunch/dinner meet for a walk. You can still chat and be sociable while also avoiding unneeded food and getting exercise.

Drink Green Tea and still be able to meet friends at café's, or read the newspaper.

Don't forget you are going 'vegetarian'. Remember the Yes & NO foods.

Many restaurants are happy to adjust a menu item slightly to keep a customer happy. Check out the menus Vegetarian section. Someone recently told me that they did not even know there was a vegetarian section on the menus as they always went for meat and since reading Daniel Diet have discovered a whole new world of recipes and they taste wonderful.

Order your meal without danger foods (e.g. chips, potato, rice etc.). It is easier to avoid it if it is not on your plate (brown rice is ok)

Ask for all dressings/sauces to be served on the side. Substitute creamy salad dressings for vinaigrette. Be aware of the hidden ingredients and sugars that can be included in many sauces.

If possible have a look at the menu online before you go out. Make note of the healthiest options or decide on what you are going to eat before you get there to avoid impulse decisions.

Avoid buffet and 'all you can eat' style restaurants. Too many temptations.

Avoid alcohol.

Q. "How Often Should I Do The Diet?"

You can do the diet as often as you wish, but I would suggest that three or four times a year would be the ideal. It's up to you to decide.

Q. "Beans and lentils (legumes) give me wind (flatulence). What can I do about this?"

Many people have difficulty digesting beans and lentils. What happens is that fermentation develops in their intestinal area, causing gas formation (sugar causes a similar reaction). To avoid the excess gas, it is wise to soak them overnight and discard the water. The soaking reduces phytic acid, an ingredient of these foods which causes 'wind' problems. For people with this problem, one or more of the following suggestions will help. Firstly, soak your lentils overnight and pour off the water next morning – don't cook them in the soaking water. Add a pinch of the Indian herb, Asa Foetida, also called Hing. It can be obtained from Indian grocery stores. Also add (to your taste), one or more of the following - anise, dill, fennel or caraway seeds – 1 teaspoon for 250 g legumes. Finally, add one to two small pieces of Kombu (a seaweed) while cooking the beans or lentils. Seaweed (kelp) is also very beneficial for weight loss and should be added to your diet, this is one way to include it. Make sure you cook them sufficiently as well. If this fails then your choice to have or not to have?

Q. "Will Daniel's Diet help if I suffer from food allergies or intolerances and what will happen if I choose to do nothing?"

Most allergies or food sensitivities come from wheat, grains, dairy, sugar, soy and junk foods. Be careful of nuts, even though they are recommended on this diet, people can be allergic to them, and you don't want to be eating too many. By going on Daniel's Diet you avoid most of the common allergens and so it will help you very much.

If you have allergies, intolerances or food sensitivities and you continue in the lifestyle you are currently in the symptoms will either remain constant or in most cases, become progressively worse or even create another symptom entirely. A continuing allergy weakens your immune system causing the environment inside your body to become susceptible to diseases. As you get older different sicknesses or symptoms usually manifest. You only have to look at the hospitals to see how overloaded they are with multiple modern disease factors. If you do this diet and continue on a moderation lifestyle you can prevent a lot of future sickness in your life. Now is the time to act. Make choices for yourself or they will be made for you. Even a moderate change will make a moderate difference. So a radical change will make a radical difference.

Q. "What if I am taking medications for serious long-term problems (e.g. diabetes, heart disease, psychiatric disorders, liver or kidney etc)?"

Do not commence Daniel's Diet without first consulting your doctor if you are on serious medication. General medications you keep taking as per normal and still go ahead with the diet. If you're in this predicament of taking medications and want to try and get off them, start thinking about what natural therapies you can use given your position. There is always something you can do to improve your health, even if you need to remain on medications. Many medications will work with natural therapies but there are a few that don't mix, so if taking medication just ask a practitioner if what you are taking is O.K.

There are many case histories of people who have changed their lifestyle and used natural therapies and, in turn their health improved to the extent that their doctors have reduced or stopped medications. Once again, it's imperative that your doctor and naturopath be consulted, because you need to work the right plan for you as an individual.

Q. "What About Exercising During Daniel's Diet?"

I suggest that in the first few days you take it very easy and just rest or walk at your leisure. Give your body a chance to put all its energy into the cleansing that's going on. Depending on how you feel, if you feel great then you might like to keep up your normal exercise regime. For those who are not feeling so good, I would recommend complete rest until the symptoms pass.

Do not start out on a huge exercise program if you're not used to it. It's wise to do all things in moderation and in their right order.

Q. "Vitamin Supplements - Can I Keep Taking Them Whilst On Daniel's Diet?"

Yes. You may continue to take vitamin, mineral and herb supplements during Daniel's Diet. Most supplements are to be taken with food, and since this is only a partial fast you are still eating. On a non-food, or water only fast you would not take them.

Q. "What About Menstruation and PMS?"

I have had numerous women say their PMS and different hormonal symptoms have improved and even disappeared after being on Daniel's Diet and changing their lifestyle. Often however it's necessary to add specific remedies to the diet to stimulate a healing response, other times just the diet and life style changes will do. So go ahead and do the diet and see what happens. I haven't seen any negative effects on menstruation. Although moods may get worse at your cycle time, if you are withdrawing from addictive foods.

Q. "What If I am already underweight? Am I able to do Daniel's diet?"

Being naturally underweight makes most overweight people very envious – but it's a very real problem to those who are too thin. In my experience, I have learnt that many thin people over eat. They are just blessed with genes that burn up fat quickly.

However, Daniel's Diet is not just about weight – it's also about detoxifying your body. Every person accumulates toxins daily because of the environment, the world in which we live and the foods we eat. Being thin does not exclude you, in fact people who can eat anything and not put on weight usually do eat wrong foods and to excess. This often means toxic overload. No matter the body shape, blood or figure type, we all need Daniel's Diet on a regular basis. For those who are very thin (underweight) and are eating regular meals; you must consider your genetic inheritance, and realize that you inherited 'thin genes' to start with.

However, what you are currently eating can also affect you. Most underweight people I see in my clinic are overeating foods that their bodies have sensitivity to, whether they realize it or not. This food sensitivity causes an internal irritation where they experience poor digestion and assimilation. Their everyday food choices, that they often believe are good for them, are actually doing the opposite. It's keeping them more underweight than the normal genetic inheritance would indicate. Usually the internal irritation causes a 'leaky gut' syndrome. Simply meaning undigested food particles are escaping back into the blood stream from your gut. This ultimately causes pressure on their immune system and allergies (sensitivities) develop and may cause your body's metabolism to speed up. This scenario places a strain on your system, which keeps you thin. By doing this diet and working out the foods that irritate your system, your body will plateau out at its optimum weight. Then you can work on a healthy regime to tone and bulk up.

Case History

An interesting example of this was an underweight patient of mine who was worried she couldn't do Daniel's Diet with the rest of her church, who were using it as a corporate partial fast. I first had to overcome the fear she had of losing more weight.

Her normal diet consisted of:
Breakfast - Cereal with milk and sugar for breakfast. Sometimes toast and jelly, a coffee with milk and 2 sugars.
Snacks - She 'just had to eat between meals' as she felt weak and irritable if she didn't. These foods were often wheat-based cookies or crackers, sweet snacks or bread.
Lunch - sandwiches
Dinner - meat and vegetables or pasta or white rice dishes, with bread. Nearly every night chocolate was eaten as sweets.

My analysis:

Lyn was on a diet far too high in carbohydrates, especially wheat (white flour).

Understand that in most people a high carbohydrate diet will cause weight gain. However for Lyn it was the opposite. She had sensitivities or allergies to grains (especially wheat) and all refined carbohydrates, she was also hypoglycemic (sugar problems) and this was why she found it so hard to change her diet.

I put Lyn on Daniel's Diet to break the sugar addiction and refined carbohydrate and grain allergy. After this diet I put her on another one high in Protein. Proteins are less inflammatory and allergenic, although some people may be allergic to eggs.

I used the Chromium and Gymnema supplement (already mentioned in chapter 9) to aid the hypoglycemia problem and also in her situation, recommended a vegetarian based high protein powder drink, mixed twice daily in half water and half coconut milk. This was to alleviate her fear of losing more weight and to support her system in the transition from her old diet to her new one.

She said withdrawals were not easy to start with but the end result was that she felt great and her weight eventually balanced out to what her genes allowed as normal. This was 6.6 pounds (3 kg) more than at the commencement, which she was happy with and enough for her to want to stay on a healthy diet.

In this case the Daniel's Diet was healthier than the original. It helped Lyn get over the fear of losing too much weight if she changed from her original diet and it set her free from an unhealthy eating cycle. Lyn was able to complete the spiritual partial fast with her church and received physical healing as well.

This is an example of modifying the diet to suit individual needs based on modern lifestyle health issues.

• You would need to consider a healthy Protein shake with the diet. Also common sense indicates that you don't eat hot foods that speed up your metabolism. Seek Naturopathic advice as there are herbs to slow the metabolism down if too high.

Q. "Can i follow daniel's diet if I am breast feeding?"
The answer to this is both 'yes' and 'no'!

The 'yes' part means you can use the Daniel's Diet as your dietary foundation or base. After all it is what we should be eating anyway, so all those vegetables, fruits and seeds will be great for the mum and baby.

However (the no part), when breast feeding you don't want to go through a sudden 'detox', as this may release toxins out of the mother and through to the baby. The mother hopefully has cut back on a lot of the harmful foods mentioned already, and if not then slowly begin to cut down over a few weeks. I suggest if you haven't already, start the Daniel's Diet, but do a modified version. This simply means adding to Daniel's Diet some good quality protein, e.g. adding daily one or more of the following; Fish, free range eggs and chicken/turkey, including a little red meat (two – three times a week). Also some whole grains in moderation.

This way you are having the best of both worlds and then when you stop breast feeding you are going to be healthier (and baby too).

Part of the 'no' factor is that you don't take any of the detox herbs when breast feeding (or if pregnant for that matter). You should be taking a multi vitamin/mineral, a probiotic and non farmed fish oil. The recommended protein shakes are also ok.

Q. "Are you allowed to eat oils on this diet?"
The old saying 'there are good oils and there are bad oils' is true. In other words – yes, oils are good for you but it will depend on which ones you use. Cold pressed oil, contained in dark glass bottles is the best and safest way to buy all oils. Here the liquid has been extracted without the use of chemicals or excess heat. Light and oxygen causes rancidity so that's why storage in dark glass is important. Most oils are preservative-free, but for anyone concerned about the oil going off (rancid), I recommend emptying two capsules of 500 IU of vitamin E oil into the bottle after opening it. Because the vitamin E's powerful antioxidant qualities will help prevent oxidization and therefore rancidity.

Remember no frying oil while on this program. But uncooked (raw) oils on your salad and vegetables are highly recommended. You can't go wrong with cold pressed Olive oil, Mustard seed oil, Flaxseed oil, Sesame oil, Coconut oil. With all oils and nuts there is the chance of rancidity especially Flaxseed oil. Always make sure that when you purchase flaxseed it is kept refrigerated at the time of buying. It's easy to test if they are rancid. Simply taste it, if the taste is bitter, it's rancid. Take it back to the shop and get a refund or another bottle. Flax seed oil is very healthy to use. It contains omega-6 and omega-9 essential fatty acids, B vitamins and some minerals. Use it raw or unheated on your salads. Olive oil has a history of use spanning thousands of years, and the Mediterranean countries that use it regularly experience lower levels of the diseases that are common in Australia/USA. Being a monounsaturated fat, and high in oleic acid, olive oil is one of the most stable oils and therefore a good choice for salads and light cooking. It can also be used as a spread instead of margarine or butter. Very high quality, organic olive oil would be the best choice with the second being extra virgin olive oil.

The safest oils you cook with after Daniel's Diet are coconut oil and olive, because of their high resistance to heat..

On Daniel's Diet I use organic olive or flaxseed oil with apple cider vinegar, garlic, cayenne pepper and other natural spices (use whatever combinations you prefer) as a salad dressing. I also use it on my steamed vegetables to enhance the taste.

Q. "Can you eat dried fruit on Daniel's diet?"
You can eat some in moderation and only if they are sun dried. You don't want to be eating sulphur dried fruit as the sulphur can cause health issues. Dried Fruit is high in sugar.

Q. "Can you Eat lots of Fruit and Lose Weight?"
Yes you can as the many of hundreds of testimonies confirm! However there are some people who may not.

There is a percentage of people who may have 'fructose intolerance'; these people will have to modify the diet to suit their specific needs.

I suggest you eat lots of variety of fruit, even if it's just for the ten days you are on this diet regime. If you are not losing weight after the ten days then this issue of fructose sugar should be considered along with other factors mentioned in my books and changes made to suit individuals. See my eBook '*5 Common Foods That Cause Bloated Stomachs and Embarrassing Flatulence.*'

However the idea of this diet is to encourage people to start eating more fruit because the statistics show the general population does not eat enough fruit. I want people to want to eat more fruit in short and long term, to get in the daily habit, eating fruit instead of modern day candy, sweets etc. This is much better for your health, weight and longevity.

Fruit has healing nutritional and cleansing factors in them, that can't be ignored, especially for detoxing. I am well aware of low and high GI (Glycemic Index) factors found in fruits. In other words – it is wise to eat low GI fruit for weight loss; on the other hand it's far better to eat fruit with high GI than it is to eat refined carbohydrates etc with high GI (I am sure you understand what I am getting at here).

I suggest you choose to eat just the low GI fruit if you are concentrating on weight loss. If you are battling on-going weight problems it's wise to know all the foods with High GI and definitely cut them down, especially the non-fruit ones. Buy or find a book in your local community Library on High/Low GI (Glycemic Index) if you are interested in pursuing this topic.

One of the wonderful things about this diet is that after you finish it – what happens or does not happen will tell a lot about your personal health status.

On average 3 pieces of fruit daily is good for you. Just use variety.
Suggestions for Low-Carbohydrate Fruits

Apples	Apricots
Blackberries	Blueberries
Cherries	Grapefruit
Limes	Lemons
Melons	Peaches

| Passion fruit | Raspberries |
| Strawberries | Mulberries – all Berries |

Q. "Rice milk - oat milk - coconut milk and soy milk - during this diet?"

No its best not to use any milk substitutes during the 10 days. If you choose to have any – coconut milk would be best. After or post diet is a different protocol.

Q. "Can you Eat 'Health Bars' on this diet?"

No! I know you probably lead a very busy life, and these so called health bars are very convenient to have on hand. It can also be confusing because they are promoted as a health food snack.

However many of these bars are so loaded with gluten, which is a highly allergenic substance for many people with sensitivities. They nearly all contain loads of sugar; therefore they aren't any better than eating a candy bar. Remember I discussed fructose corn syrup (HFCS). This chemically-converted, non-natural, corn-based sweetener can have negative effects on health. This form of Fructose is metabolized to fat more than other sugars, making it clearly fat-promoting. Other bars contain the artificial sugars also mentioned previously.

Post Daniel's Diet you can look for a 'top' quality, dense protein and gluten free Bar if you need to, (email me if you need help).

Q. "Is it Wise to be a vegetarian in the Long Term?"

The answer is both yes and no!

You can CHOOSE to be a vegetarian if that is what you want; however, you must do some due diligence and do it properly. You should know what you are doing, nutritionally wise, as it is difficult to find vitamin B12, iron, amino acids and complete protein in the vegetables. Meat on the other hand is an easy way to ingest these nutrients.

Most vegetarians eat far too much refined carbs, dairy food and sugar (to compensate for the lack of good quality protein), which is unhealthy.

Q. Daniel's diet is a Vegan Diet for a short time of 10 days.

Vegans are those who eat NO animal product at all, including no eggs, milk and cheese.

Therefore it's very much a personal decision but you must have the knowledge to make an informed choice on what is the best lifestyle and diet to your health and longevity.

Personally I have been a vegan for many years but changed a few years ago.

Now I eat fish (ones with scales only) plenty of fruits, nuts, seeds, vegetables and herbs. I personally eat red meat once or twice a week and chicken (or turkey) once per week. Eggs I have three times a week and I only eat high quality breads, never white or commercial ones. I drink only filtered water and exercise daily.

However I often 'go' Vegetarian for a 'season' and follow my Daniel's diet when I feel I should. E.g. If I feel any kind of tiredness or ill health symptoms trying to get hold of me. I do it to freshen up mentally and physically if I need to. I also believe in the power of fasting for health and spiritual growth.

Contraindications to doing this diet

Some diseases and conditions will prevent people from following this diet. These illnesses and physical states include:

- Diabetes
- Epilepsy
- Pregnancy
- Serious heart disease
- Severe anemia
- anyone on psychiatric medication
- Anyone physically or emotionally fragile or run down

There is, however, no need for anyone to miss out on improving his or her health through dietary change. All you have to do is adjust the foundation of this diet to suit your individual situation. For example, if you are physically run down and weak, start by doing this diet for one or two days at a time and as you improve build up to three or four days until you can manage what is beneficial to you. You can do what I call a modified Daniel's Diet. This means the foundation of your eating is what you have learnt in this book but you simply add some other healthy choices to it. Examples add fish, eggs, some whole grains. If we use common sense and wisdom we can always improve our health situation.

I am encouraging Wisdom For Health so if you are in any of these categories, are taking strong medication, or are unsure, please consult a medical practitioner or naturopath before starting Daniel's Diet.

I believe that taking responsibility for our own health, together with herbs, medicine and prayer, will always give hope and offer the potential to be healed.

There are many testimonies from people who have been healed of various diseases by following a strict healthy lifestyle program. Never give up if you are in ill health. "Seek and you shall find. Knock and the door will be open to you."(Matthew 7:7) In my clinic it's the people who stick with my treatments, the ones who continue over a period of time and don't give up who will always get the results they are aiming for.

This book will start the process of health and healing for you. If you follow God's Principles for Health, you are allowing your body to heal itself. It's been designed that way. The only criteria being that you have to do it.

There are no short cuts to long-term health and weight loss. You have to take responsibility for it. Go on and start now.

PART SIX

EXAMPLE RECIPES:

CHAPTER NINETEEN

RECIPE EXAMPLES

R ecipe examples taken from my book 'The Daniel's Way Recipe Guide': to help you start the diet and give ideas on vegetarian food that is very 'yummy'. The new recipe book is available in Kindle, EBook, or Paperback, from my web site or Amazon.com.

BREAKFAST

Millet Porridge
Ingredients
1 cup hulled millet
3 cups water
Berries to taste
Any low GI fruit to your taste
Add some pumpkin seeds or Chia, sesame, flax seeds or even a tablespoon of lecithin granules.

Millet is a grain that is gluten-free. It is alkaline and easy to digest and as a bonus has good protein content. Eat 2/3 of a small breakfast bowl per meal.

Preparation Method
Boil the water then add the millet. Simmer for 15-20 minutes or until millet is soft. It forms a mucilaginous texture when cooked which act as an intestinal lubricant and benefits your 'tummy'.
If the texture becomes 'gluggy', strain it under running water.

Fruit Porridge

Made from fresh fruit, it is beautifully sweet and light and makes a delicious dessert as well as a breakfast dish. You can include the prune recipe with this and any fruit breakfasts.

1 pear (or strawberries, apple etc.)
1/4 cup pumpkin seeds and/or pine and Brazil nuts
1/2 ripe banana or ¼ cup of prunes
2 tbsp LSA (linseed, sunflower seeds and almonds; found at most health and retail stores)

Mince the seeds and nuts together in the food processor until they are well chopped. Then add the rest of the ingredients until smooth. Add water or coconut milk to make 'porridge'.

MORNING AND AFTERNOON TEA

DIPS

Great to have with sliced carrot, beans, celery and zucchini. This is a good idea if entertaining or socializing.

Ground Chick Pea Dip

Ingredients
125 g dried chick peas
80g toasted sesame seeds
4 tbsp chopped oregano, basil, or other herbs in season
1-2 cloves garlic
2 cups veggie stock
1 tbsp lime juice
3 tbsp red onion, chopped
1 tsp Dijon mustard
pinch Himalayan salt

Preparation Method

Grind the chick peas in a blender to a powder like cornmeal. Cook in the boiling stock for about 10 minutes, constantly stirring. Let cool, and mix with the rest of the ingredients. Serve as a dip with baby carrots, beans, celery and zucchini

Guacamole

Ingredients

1 avocado

1 tsp red onion, finely chopped

1 medium tomato

1 tbsp fresh lemon juice

Pinch Celtic salt

Black pepper

Splash of tamari

Optional: pinch of cayenne, or ½ tsp turmeric

Preparation Method

Blend in a food processor. Or mash the avocado with a fork, add onion, tomatoes and seasonings and mix well.

LUNCH

SALAD RECIPES
Rainbow Salad

I encourage you to use your imagination and mix any combination and amount to suit your appetite and taste. Make it an enjoyable challenge to mix and match different colours. Remember to wash your vegetables.

Ingredients

- yellow or red capsicum, asparagus, celery, cucumber
- red cabbage, eggplant, parsley, onion
- spinach, comfrey, broccoli, baby peas

- tender carrots, alfalfa sprouts, lettuce, endive
- turnip, fennel, cauliflower, parsley
- squash, snow peas, beetroot, tomato

Philip's Rainbow Salad
Ingredients
- asparagus, celery, snow peas, onion
- beetroot, tomatoes, mixed lettuce, avocado
- walnuts, yellow capsicum, red/purple cabbage, cauliflower

Preparation Method
Chop or grate whatever amount you need for the meal. Drizzle with a dressing of olive oil, garlic and apple cider vinegar or lemon juice, with a pinch of turmeric and cayenne.

Grilled Sweet Potato with Coriander Pesto and Salad
Ingredients
1 kg of sweet potato, peeled, marinated in a cup of water with the 3 tbs. lemon juice
1 bunch fresh asparagus steamed until tender
1 medium red capsicum quartered and char grilled and peeled and cut into cubes
1 small Lebanese cucumber cut into strips
160 g salad greens
Marinate 1 cm thick sweet potato slices for 5 minutes. Dry and grill under a low grill setting with a little oil.
Turn them and make sure the brown but don't burn

Preparation Method
Gently toast 100 grams pine nuts and blend together in a food processor
With ½ to a whole red chilli - remember some like it hot!!
2 cloves of Garlic minced

1 large bunch of coriander with the stems and roots
2 tablespoon of lime juice
2 tablespoon Olive oil
Sea salt to taste
Arrange the veggies and salad greens on a platter, and serve the sweet potato with the coriander pesto

Philip's Favourite Salad Dressing
Ingredients
1 garlic clove
2 tablespoons squeeze lemon juice
1 tablespoon cold pressed olive oil or flaxseed oil
Pinch turmeric
Other herbs to taste

Preparation Method
Crush garlic clove. Squeeze lemon and to it garlic, oil and herbs to taste.
Adjust amounts of these ingredients to suit your salad size and taste. You will need to make a healthy dressing to make your salads more tasty and interesting.

Salads and Soups can be eaten for lunch and/or dinner.

Traditionally Cooked Foods That Can Be Eaten Raw:
Beetroot (beet), pumpkin, cauliflower and broccoli can be shredded and eaten raw if mixed with a suitable dressing such as lemon juice, apple cider vinegar, herbs and olive oil.

Various herbs such as chilli, garlic, rosemary, bay leaves, etc. can be added for different flavours. Artichokes, asparagus, cauliflower, broccoli, young beans and peas can also be eaten raw. Sprouted peas, beans, chick peas, lentils, sunflower seeds, etc. are also delicious with a dressing.

Soup

Lentil & Spinach Soup

Recipe courtesy Genevieve Baster-Sallen

½ packet sprouted lentils or ¼ cup raw lentils

8-12 spinach leaves

1 cup carrot

½ cup sweet potato

¼ brown onion

¼ tsp cumin

1 tsp dried herbs

1½ cups water

1 clove garlic

Preparation Method

If using raw lentils, place in a large pot of water and cook uncovered for 1 hour. Rinse and drain well.

In another saucepan add the water, onion, herbs, cumin, carrots, and sweet potato. Simmer for 10–15 minutes. Add the lentils.

Gently tear the spinach leaves into bite-size pieces and stir through the soup.

Blend well in a blender or food processor and serve with a salad.

DINNER

Brown Rice with an Italian flavour

Ingredients

3 cups of cooked brown short grain rice

1 onion chopped

1 dessertspoon lime zest

2 small cloves of garlic minced

½ cup toasted slivered almonds
½ cup sundried tomatoes sliced fine
½ cup sliced black olives
½ cup of chopped fresh basil
½ cup of chopped flat leaf parsley
Sauté the onions and garlic in a little olive oil until soft
Add the garlic and zest stirring for a minute or so
Stir in the cooked rice and heat through.

Now mix the Dressing ingredients in a jar,
3 tablespoons of lime juice
1 tablespoon of white balsamic vinegar
Two cloves of garlic crushed
½ teaspoon of Dijon mustard
teaspoons of veggie stock and one tablespoon of olive oil

Preparation Method
Assemble the Salad by mixing the dressing into the rice with the herbs and the rest of the ingredients.
Adjust the seasoning add salt to taste

Chick Pea Curry
Ingredients
1 onion, chopped
1 leek
2 cloves garlic
1 tsp curry paste
Cumin, black pepper, paprika to taste
1 cup vegetable stock
1 cup cooked chick peas
3 large carrots, chopped
1 cup cauliflower pieces
1/3 fresh pineapple pieces

½ cup cashews (mixed with cooked meal)

Preparation Method

Cook together onion, leek and garlic in a little oil or water. Add curry paste and seasonings, cook for 1 minute. Add veggie stock and chick peas, carrots and cauliflower. Simmer till cooked about ½ hour. Then add pineapple pieces, and cashews. Allow to stand for about ½ hour for flavours to mingle.

Serve with Brown Rice. (Rice cooked in turmeric and mixed with cooked lentils is very good.)

PART SEVEN

TESTIMONIES

CHAPTER TWENTY

TESTIMONIES

Testimonies from people all over the world who have followed this books teaching:

Most of the following testimonies are quotes from emails or letters sent to me. I have many more from seminars and Ministry at churches. Some are so profound that you can only say – 'Praise be to Jesus'. I have tested this diet plan for many years and have had so much success with it that I encourage you with these real testimonies; that you can overcome any health problems as these people have. I also encourage you that our Heavenly Father does care about your health and that He does have a natural Health Plan for you to follow.

This book was first released in Australia as 'Daniel's Diet'; which is a best seller and award winning published book. 'Daniel's Way to Lose Weight' is a new and improved version and the name has been changed to launch it worldwide in 2017.

When the testimonies talk of Daniel's diet it is this book that you are reading now they are referring to not other books with similar names.

Success Stories
See more on video testimonies click the link down below
http://www.youtube.com/user/danielsdetox?feature=mhee

Hello Philip - I know that the Holy Spirit led me to your book; there was no other way to describe it. Before I started Daniels Way to Weight loss, I was in a lot of pain and I wasn't able to walk my dog on the local walking trail without stopping at the first public seat about half a kilometre from my home where he could run leash free. The pain in my knees/hip was so bad that I had to sit for at least ten minutes before making my way home again. Since Christmas shopping got in the way I haven't walked the dog for some time (I could shop or walk the dog, not both). I waited for three days into the diet before I decided to walk the dog. The first day I sat for a minute at the most before getting up and going a little further, the next day I didn't bother with my old seat, I felt so good and just walked; each day has been a little further. This morning I walked further still and afterwards went shopping with my niece, to both ends of the shopping centre. As I said earlier, in the past this was impossible, I could go shopping or take the dog out, not both. There is barely any pain left now, I know in time and with God's grace, it will completely go. I also lost 2kg and 3.5 cm off my waist.

From Latysha:
Dear Philip, I am writing from USA to thank you for changing my life! I followed your diet as you advised wanting to "lose weight quickly before Christmas". I "did" the diet and lost quite a few inches (centimetres) and I have lost 11 pounds (5kg) all up and fit into all my old clothes.

From Monica:
Lost 49 pounds (22 kg) and that's not all - "By following the 10 day diet plan and then continuing on with your low Carb' diet ('The 6 Week Low Carb Diet'). I have lost 49 pounds over 3 months. Not only that but my Doctor has reduced my blood pressure medication by three quarters and my cholesterol has come down from 6.5 to 4.

From David:
I feel 100% better. I still feel a little tired, but nothing like I used to feel. I feel more energized. My wife has been really encouraged because my jerky/twitchy legs and continuous moving in my sleep has stopped; I am very still at night now. I now drink 2 quarts of water daily. I have not

had a head ache worth mentioning since I started on the diet and supplements, nor since I came off them. So thank you Philip.

These are my results so far…

1. Sleep improved 100%
2. Do not move like a trapeze artist at night
3. My wife is sleeping well most nights now since I have been on this diet
4. Wind/flatulence has decreased dramatically
5. My sleep talking is less but clearer!
6. No headaches in 3 weeks
7. I have lost weight
8. I do not have a bloated stomach anymore
9. I have a huge amount of energy now
10. I wake up in the morning refreshed
11. I can go to bed much later now with no obvious negativity as a result
12. Waking up on weekends alert and refreshed after a little lie in - this rarely occurred before
13. Body feels lighter
14. I do not feel tense in the body
15. I do not feel the pressure in my veins for caffeine
16. I do not feel anxiety
17. I do not feel stressed
18. I feel fresh and alert through the day
19. I have a better appetite
20. My body is more flexible
21. I have not bitten my nails in 3 weeks
22. General feeling of well-being
23. Much more clearer in my thinking
24. My body seems to be healing – I have had issues with my back which seems to be getting much better
25. I am more tolerant.

So, as you can see it is working somewhat! Thanks a million Philip.

From Gemmy:

I am amazed to find that Daniel's diet does actually work. Take this from someone with a slow metabolism, who doesn't have time for regular exercise due to work commitments. Someone who was beginning to believe that she had an eating disorder due to uncontrollable binge eating, and who has tried nearly every diet I have come across.

I'm beginning to feel less stressed and have fewer hot flushes. I think more clearly and sleep better, have had very few urges to binge eat, and am not hungry at all It is also not an expensive diet to do, which is fantastic, considering the amount of money I have wasted over the years.

I have now lost 9.2 pounds (4.2kg) over the ten days of the diet. When you think that during my other diet attempts where overall I gained weight instead of losing it, I am thrilled.

From Molly:

Since starting I lost 14 pounds and several inches off my waist. Which is fine with me - and yes!... I can do all things through Christ who strengthens me.

From Anonymous:

Dear Philip, I have just completed your detox diet, and can't believe I did it. I feel sooooo renewed & sooooooo in control of my life. I did not realize the hold coffee had over me. You warned of detoxing effects but 'wow' is all I cansay. I started your detox as suggested, lowering certain foods 2 weeks prior to the actual detox. After reading your comments on coffee, I knew I had to start there. So in the first week, I cut my first cup per day out, which was fine & then completely in the 2nd week. Here's where it all happened... by 10.00am without coffee, I had a headache, by 3.00 pm I was wondering if it was all worth it, but having come so far, I was determined to continue. Within the next hour my headache turned into the worst migraine I have had in years (I have suffered migraines for many years). 2 days later I recovered, realizing how severe my coffee addiction had been and how it was controlling my life. I can't believe that I am not craving at all now (actually giving up coffee altogether). Since the diet I have lost the cravings. It's all so amazing. My husband is also inspired by what I have just done, so he is joining me on our good healthy eating plan. A huge 'thank you' for speaking the truth into our lives & for sharing your knowledge.

From Tammy:
My mother decided after reading your book that she would go off coffee first then she would begin the ten day detox. She suffered headaches for three days just giving up the coffee. By the seventh day of the detox my mother was glowing. She was so excited that for the first time in 11 years she slept the whole night through and when she woke up she was finished sleeping and sprung out of bed with renewed energy. Her skin changed and the whites of her eyes were brighter. She said she has never felt as good as she did being on that detox.

Stories from friends:
Another story was a friend's husband who suffered diabetes and obesity. He read the book and changed his lifestyle losing 55 pounds (25 kilos) to date and his character change was most noticeable. So much more positive, not reactive – he seemed like a new man.

***

My good friend suffers asthma daily and after 7 days on this diet plan she enjoyed the realization that she didn't require her asthma spray all day and for the next week. Allergies disappeared and a skin change occurred. **PLUS:** After three short weeks of following your diet recommendations, my son lost 3.5 inches (9 cm) in the waist, stopped sweating when he ate and yes… The pimple patches disappeared.

That week I received a letter from his teacher via email telling me that DJ had really turned a corner as he had finished every task, was not in trouble for talking and seemed very calm and relaxed! He then said…

whatever you're doing… keep it up!

From Livy:
Philip- I'm on your diet, now today is my 10th day and I lost 12lbs. hallelujah!

From Winnie:
I was engrossed in your book again last night and I have come to the conclusion it is not just a book but a wonderful investment. I am so glad I found it and I will certainly be buying more copies for my friends with the hope they will find it as beneficial as myself.

From Josie:
Hi Philip, on the 9th day of your detox diet, feeling fantastic - lost 13 pounds (6kgs). Looking forward to reading your new lifestyle book.

From Tammy:
"I have tried several weight-loss associations, clubs, etc. and the weight I lost wasn't permanent. I heard about Philip's ministry meetings and attended them regularly for one school term. My life started to change dramatically, right from the first lecture.

Habitual eating for comfort and loneliness just started losing its hold over me. I finally realized chocolate is not a friend. The last time I ate it I noticed I got a real 'high' or 'upper,' then shortly after that, I got emotionally low, grumpy and depressed which lasted for the rest of the day. This affected my entire family. I have learnt 'you are what you eat,' and I can control my moods, emotions, health and myself - by eating properly.

Since attending the teachings, I find it a lot easier to change my eating habits and cooking styles. It works. Thanks Philip."

From Ethan:
I live in Sydney Australia. I read your "Daniel's Diet." It is the best diet book I have ever read. Many thanks!

From Barbara:

Hi Philip - I just wanted to let you know that a group of us are doing your 10 day Diet again starting today! After getting one of my friends onto it some months ago...she has organized about 10 of us to do a group effort! I thought it might be encouraging for you to know what goes on every so often! Word of mouth has now got out because of the marvelous results and our group is growing so much that the church we belong to is going to send you an invite to come and teach a seminar with us. We are all so much looking forward to that – we pray that you will come.

From Bianca:

I was desperate for help – I had shooting pains to my heart. I was tired and listless, no energy – Finding it hard to keep up with chores and walking the dog. It took every bit of will power & determination to walk up the steps at my Church. I am classed as Diabetic (type 2). I had a massive heart attack... and triple bypass some years ago. I am very overweight and all my joints ache. 2 years ago I had shingles, and was vomiting regularly. I was told I had high acid levels, and there was a lot of pressure on my heart. So - I started Daniel's Diet.... After four days on the detox... my joints freed up for the first time for years I could exercise a little bit (tears of joy flowed). In 4 days I lost 9 pounds (4 kilos), my bowels started working properly for the first time in years. After 21 days of detox I had lost 17 and a half pounds (8 kilos) and was starting to feel healthy for the first time in many years. My energy was increasing day by day; I was more awake and alert and can read the bible more without nodding off to sleep or losing concentration. My sugar (diabetes) levels were reading at 15 – Progressively they have come down to 5, Praise Jesus. The pain in my chest has gone now and all signs of shingles.

From Sue-Anne:

Hi Philip I have been so busy today but needed to tell you that I've experienced significant ongoing healing since starting Daniel's Diet, it started after I read all the daily prayers you suggested in the book..... I started feeling better and better and more alive. I know the food addictions are all gone. Today nearly everywhere I went people complimented me saying I looked, gorgeous or pretty or glowing etc and I was amazed. I could even feel the 'fog' at the front of my forehead/brain area disappearing. I feel really blessed and thankful, instead of feeling anger I feel only loving.

From 'D:

Dear Philip, Hi my name is D... and I have been on Daniel's diet several times and have been very successful in losing weight and also detoxing from certain things. I felt very well in mind and body. The longest time I did it for was 30 days and the results were amazing. Everybody who saw me was amazed at how well I looked. I have recommended your book to many people.

From Pippa:

Dear Brother in Christ! Just a brief background on me, I am 25yr old female, small build - 5 feet 2 inches ... 2 years ago I was struggling with Anorexia - weighing in at only 39kg. I was moody, depressed - even had thoughts of suicide. I purchased your book, Daniel's Diet and almost immediately started the 10 day detox. MY MAIN problem was I had developed an obsession with binge eating breakfast cereals. HOWEVER - in 3.5 months I had gained 11-13 pounds (5-6kg). FRIGHTENING! Amazing! I thought that crazy - how could that be when I was eating 'healthy'? I have since learned - from your fantastic book - I was overloading in refined carbohydrates and I was having far too much sugar as well. I possibly also have intolerance to gluten. So when I read in your book NO CEREAL allowed on the Daniel Diet I knew that was my big give up thing! It really has helped me to get back on track with my eating – thanks so much.

From Teresa:

After completing the 10 days I not only feel SO much better - it's a wonderful feeling. On top of that already more than beneficial outcome - I felt SO ALIVE! Truly -wonderful. AND - as an added bonus I found after 10 days I was back to my ideal weight

From Lisa:

I am not overweight -but could see the benefit of doing Daniel's diet and at the end of the 10 days I could have run a marathon...I felt the fittest I had ever been and I have beaten my addiction I have completely come of sugar, no cravings - I have done it. Praise the Lord. Thanks Philip

From Pamela:

Well the benefits of concluding "Daniel's Diet" for me are:

* Weight loss - don't know how much 'cos' I never weigh myself but its visible and all my clothes are looser!
* My eczema has cleared up - no itching at all
* My skin is clearer
* My mind is clearer
* I sleep soundly
* My mood is excellent
* Not hungry no hunger pangs or cravings for a coffee etc.
  - Thanks

From Jan:

After completing the 10 day Daniel's Diet I reintroduced bread back into my diet and discovered it was the culprit for giving me long term bloated feeling and severe stomach pain. A lesson learnt.

From Wendy:

Hello Philip, Re: my Thyroid.

You will be interested to know that during the 10 days of detox, my normally erratic thyroid gland completely stabilized. I had previously undertaken measures to manage this such as cutting out coffee completely and regular exercise. However, every now and again, it would go over or under active with no indication as to why. I conclude now that the caffeine in chocolate is enough set my thyroid off on a 'spin' as the major deviation from my diet was chocolate; (Quite a lot of it considering my 10 days without it!) My skin was also very clear during the 10 days and my concentration heightened. I lost weight as well. Not sure how much but enough to make my jeans very baggy!! In short, the diet was very effective for me and I plan to do it every 3 months as you suggest. So thank you!

From Chloe:

Dear Philip – as a result of reading your book my best friend has turned back to God (and lost some weight). Bless you CL.

From Wayne:

You came to our church and talked on health and Daniels's Way to losing weight. I immediately gave up all dairy products. Result; In the past I always got recurring colds – no more. I suffered sinus and mucus problems for many years – no more. As a bonus my skin improved.

From Elle (15 years old):

"I was very overweight and couldn't seem to lose it. I felt bloated and 'puffy' as well as having no energy. Due to all this I was lacking in confidence and had a poor self-image. Philip explained Daniel's Diet to me and I committed to following it. In 10 days I lost 22 pounds (10 kg). I was feeling so good I continued on following the moderation diet plan and lost 55 pounds (25 kg) in 3 months and regained all my energy and self-esteem. My Mum is so impressed she is now following the diet."

From Cal (60 years old):

"I have just finished the ten days on Daniel's Diet and for the first time in years I can bend over and cut my toe nails. I can also put my socks on without grunting, puffing and discomfort. My pot belly is shrinking."

From Cathy:

"The best thing about doing the Daniel's Diet is that not only did I lose weight but after the diet I found I had broken the habit of eating candy (sweets) every day. I no longer get recurring colds. I also seem to cope with work pressure a lot better."

From Bill:

"I weighed 12 stone (168 pounds) when I first got married. I remained at that weight for 6 months, then, subtly things slowly changed. I started to drink a little extra beer, this seemed to increase my appetite and so slowly, I started to eat more. At this time, I was content in my marriage and this contentment seemed to draw me into eating more often than usual and my exercise decreased. To make it worse, the foods I chose were sweet sugary foods, and the quick and easy, fast food variety. Sadly, after a few years, my marriage failed and the pain, stress and trauma led me to comfort eating. My weight went to 190 pounds. Then, before I knew it, I was 225 pounds. I was so overweight my work place sent me for a medical checkup. I had high blood pressure and high cholesterol and they told me I must lose weight. I tried their diets and many others over the years. Some worked for a while, others made me feel sick. But none really worked long term. Two years later I was a whopping 244 pounds. With the weight came numerous symptoms of ill health, my confidence dropped, I felt depressed and using public transport was a problem due to my size. During this time, I had become a committed Christian and for some time had been praying and asking God for help but nothing seemed to happen. I kept praying and then one day, HJ, a Christian friend, came over to visit me. She was quite excited about a Christian teaching and weight loss meeting she was attending. She brought me a copy of Philip Bridgeman's 'Daniel's Diet'. Finally, I could see the answer to my prayer. Here was a diet plan I could believe in and understand. Now it was time for me to put my faith into action and follow the directions. The first 5 days of Daniel's Diet with all the withdrawal symptoms were very difficult. However, Philip warns about this in the book and I knew it would be only for a few days and worth it. Toward the end of the ten days, I was losing weight but I was also starting to feel much healthier. Because I was so very overweight and toxic, I asked Philip if I could stay on the diet longer. I continued the detox for 20 more days under his supervision. I felt so good after the 30 days. By this time I had lost so much weight that I decided to follow Philip's Moderation Diet and over the next 12 months not only lost all my bad health symptoms but also reached my goal weight of 176 pounds. I had lost 68 pounds."

From RC:

Many thanks for your lovely book. I was on your Daniel's diet detox program in December; it changed my life and I gave my book to my mom's friend, who could not stop reading it when I showed it to her one night in South Africa. Can you post me another copy of your book as I want to go on the detox program again? I have stopped eating gluten, drink one cup of coffee a week, as a treat - like you suggested. I even eat beetroot every day, and am just so much more aware of what I eat and how it affects me. Your book was just so refreshing because it cuts through all the modern day psycho-babble, "I-can-do-it", 'it's-my-mom's-fault-that-I-eat-too-much', and just boldly and courageously presents the facts, simple and straightforward, like all truths in God's word. I know you must get this a lot, but thank you so much! May God bless every person who reads it and all your days.

From Marlene:
"This Diet Helped Me Fall Pregnant"

I'm a professional woman in my early 30's. My husband and I had been trying for a baby for a couple of years. Philip was recommended to me by a friend, so I booked a consultation with him. He told me he didn't want me to fall pregnant for a couple of months – until I had detoxified my system. I did the pre Daniel's Diet for 2 weeks and then the Daniel's Diet for 10 days. I felt really good after this time and since I had lost weight I continued on the moderation diet taking some specific herbs and minerals/vitamins. It took only 3 months and I fell pregnant. I am convinced it was the Daniel's Diet that allowed my body to balance itself internally and I now have a little baby girl to prove it.

From Anonymous:

'The proof is in the pudding' - My excuse for being overweight had always been, 'it's in the genes.'

Following the birth of my third child I weighed 201 pounds and was starting to experience some serious health problems because of the weight and my diet. I had my gall bladder removed just a few months before I was asked to read Philip's draft for his new book, 'Daniel's Diet'. The need for change was already evident in my life. Until now, I had not had the motivation or the real desire to do something about it. But reading the book inspired me to trial the diet. I was, after all, curious to see whether it did what Philip claimed it would. Not only that, but my husband, also agreed to give it a go. This was a miracle in itself if you ask me.

I started the 10 days determined that no matter how hard it got I would stick to it and amazingly, I did. By the end of the 10 days I was feeling fitter, more motivated, and full of energy and my concentration was a lot sharper. You see, while you are on 'Daniel's Diet' you are only prohibited in eating those things that are going to cause you harm. You can still eat as many of the right foods as you need to satisfy your hunger. I became used to not eating heavy type foods and I could begin to feel my stomach shrinking which was a great feeling and encouraging.

Suffice to say, I was amazed at how good I felt and how low a priority food became in my thinking and in my life. Previously it had been an idol. My husband and I managed to lose approximately a pound a day whilst on the diet. I think it is the miracle of seeing that much weight, literally drop off. That is so encouraging. I have always felt the enormous responsibility I have towards my children, to raise them in such a way as to make them happy and healthy. Diet is an area where I have had much guilt. I can now look forward to training my children to eat properly, as they can now see me demonstrating to them 'proper' and responsible eating habits.

From Lois:

Lost 44 pounds (An extract from a letter she sent to me)

"I used to eat out of frustration, anxiety and depression. I had become a glutton and had a whole list of physical symptoms of ill health.

Your teachings on looking after the temple of the Holy Spirit (my body) and emotional eating set my mind free. I was able to complete the 10 days of Daniel's Diet. The first few days were difficult for me as I had withdrawal symptoms of headaches and generally felt 'lousy.' I was continually feeling hungry and craved all the junk food I had previously been eating. Prayer was a big help at this time and being determined to follow God's plan, knowing that He wanted me to be healthy, pulled me through.

However, after 10 days on the diet I was feeling so much better that I continued on a modified vegetarian diet for 5 months and lost over 44 pounds. Thanks to you I now understand how to choose food that is right for my body. I take the nutrient supplements you recommended and I no longer crave fatty, salty and sweet foods. Not only that but my last medical check showed that nearly all my gallstones had dissolved, and almost all the other illnesses and symptoms I had disappeared too.

Interestingly, I am also much more emotionally stable as well. Thank you so very much Philip and keep spreading the message of health and healing."

CHAPTER TWENTY ONE

WHAT PEOPLE ARE SAYING ABOUT 'GODS WAY TO WEIGHT LOSS' (DANIEL'S DIET...)

"Philip has written two books entitled *'Daniel's Diet' – the 10 day Weight Loss & Detox Diet'* and *'Daniel's Diet Lifestyle'*. I fully recommend these books. Philip understands the significance of proper nutrition and this book will give practical help in how to apply these principles to your life."

Rev Dr Margaret Court (Ao, MBE, Phd LLB Hon)

"I invited Philip Bridgeman to my Church to teach us about partial fasting and Daniel's Detox. I wanted my congregation to understand the spiritual and practical perspective, so that we could wisely undertake the fast. The teaching was excellent and the results of Daniel's Detox so profound, that we invited Philip back again for a Daniel's Detox testimony night. We were inundated with people wanting to speak. People were so impressed with great results they had received from the diet that we spent the whole night letting them give their verbal testimony to the fact - my wife and I included. I recommend Philip to any Church or group to hear his teaching and encourage anyone to do the diet."

Pastor Claude Carrelo, River of Life Church

"This book is educational, empowering, easy to understand, making the diet very achievable."

Liz Gillman, N.D. Naturopath (Dip Nat Med)

"The story of Daniel's Detox as described in Daniel chapter one, teaches us profound Biblical dietary and health principles. This book explores the same principles in an easy to read, modern manner in great detail. If we want to be healthy and happy, begin here with this book."

Pastor James Fitzsimmons,
Seventh Day Adventist Church

"By using the principles set out in Daniel's Detox, I have personally overcome a health issue I 'was' facing. I most strongly endorse Philip and his book."

Pastor Russell Sage, Ministries International

"This is an amazing detailed, yet simple diet that follows solid Biblical precepts. Philip goes into the 'truth' that sets one free – the truth that everyone is a spirit, living in a body dominated by the soulish realm of the mind, will and emotions. He skillfully explains the types of 'foods' for all three areas that provides the necessary fuel for the person to be made whole. By so doing, it enables the reader to be able to change and overcome things in their life that before they found too difficult. This provides a diet and health principles that can literally change your life. This book gives answers to health and losing weight, by expanding on biblical principles. It is unique in this sense and by looking at spirit, soul and body it caters for every individual needs.

I highly recommend this book and it's common sense approach will appeal to all. It also has huge potential as an evangelical tool to approach friends, neighbors and relatives to introduce them to not only health of the body but to Jesus, and their spiritual side."

Rev Barbara Oldfield-Bentley, Victory Life Church

REFERENCES

Welcome to 'Daniels Way' - to Weight Loss

1. Tremblay A. Dietary fat and body weight set point. Nutr Rev, 2004; 62[7]:s75-77. Obese have higher toxin levels.
2. Dawson-Hughes B et al. Alkaline Diets favour lean tissue mass in older adults. AMJ. Clinical. Nutrition. 2008:87:662-5.

CHAPTER 2

1. Sydney Morning Herald. http:www.smh.com.au/lifestyle/wellbeing/obesity-is-now-more-deadly-than-smoking-20100408-rv5l.html
2. (As listed by AC Nielson in 1999)
3. The Western Australian Tuesday, September 27, 2016, news p.3.
4. From The Medscape Journal of Medicine: Fruit and Vegetable Intake Among Adolescents and Adults in the United States: Percentage Meeting Individualized Recommendations. Posted 01/26/2009. Joel Kimmons, PhD; Cathleen Gillespie, MS; Jennifer Seymour, PhD; Mary Serdula, MD; Heidi Michels Blanck, PhD

CHAPTER 5

1. Maki KC, Reeves MS et al. Green tea catechin consumption enhances exercise-induced abdominal fat loss in overweight and obese adults. Nutrition; 2009 Feb; 1 39 [2]: 264-70
2. Auvichayapat P, et al. Effectiveness of green tea on weight reduction in obese Thais: A randomized, controlled trial. Physiol behave. 2008 Feb 27; 93[3]: 486-91.

CHAPTER 9:

- Eurekalert December 16, 2008
- Khan N, Mukhtar H.Cancer and metastasis: prevention and treatment by green tea. Cancer Metastasis Rev. 2010 Sep; 29[3]:435-45. Review.
- Liang G, Tang A, Lin X, Li L, Zhang S, Huang Z, Tang H, Li QQ. Green Tea catechins augment the antitumor activity of doxorubicin in an in vivo mouse model for chemoresistant liver cancer. Int J Oncol. 2010 Jul: 37[1]:111-23.
- Journal of the National Cancer Institute (1997;89(24):1881-1886)
- European Journal of Clinical Nutrition August, 2000; 54:618-625.
- The Lancet March 10, 2001; 357:732, 746-751
- Journal of Agricultural and Food Chemistry May 11, 2011; 59[9]:5125-32
- Michaelsson K, Wolk A, Langenskiold S, et al. Milk intake and risk of mortality and fractures in women and men: cohort studies. Bmj 2014; 349: g6015.
- Castelo-Branco C, Pons f, Vicente JJ, Sanjuan A, Vanrell JA, Preventing postmenopausal bone loss with osseinhydroxyapatite compounds. Result of a two- year, prospective trial. J Reprod Med 1999; 44[7]:601-5.
- Plus; Fernandez-Pareja et al. Prevention of Osteoporosis: Four-Year Follow- Up of a Cohort of Postmenopausal Women Treated with an Ossein-Hydroxyapatite Compound. Clin. Drug Investig. 2007; 27[4]:227-232
- Medical News Today May 8, 2013
- "Table 52 – High fructose corn syrup: estimated number of per capita calories consumed daily, by calendar year.' Ers.usda.gov/briefing/sugar/data.htm
- Washington Post January 26, 2009
- Swithers, S.E. Behavioral Neuroscience, February 2008; online edition.
- A study at the University of Texas Health Science Center in San Antonio

CHAPTER 10:

- Verma SP, Goldin BR, Lin PS. The inhibition of the oestrogenic effects of pesticides and environmental chemicals by curcumin and isoflavonoids. Environ Health Perspect. 1998 Dec; 106 [12]: 807-12

- Zhou QM. Curcumin enhanced antiproliferative effect of mitomycin C in human breast cancer MCF-7 cells in vivo.Acta Pharmacol Sin. 2011 Nov;32[11]:1402.10

- Asami DK, et al. Comparison of the total phenolic and ascorbic acid content of freeze-dried and air-dried marionberry, starberry and corn grown using conventional, organic, and sustainable agricultural practices. J Agric Food Chem. 2003 Feb. 26; 51 [5]:1237-41

- World's Healthiest Foods, Watermelon

- Jurenka JS. Therapeutic applications of pomegranate (Punica granatum L.): a review. Altern Med Rev. 2008 Jun; 13 [2]:128-44

- Dr Irving Fisher, Yale University Meat vs. Vegetables 2000. The Wellspring Publishers.

ACKNOWLEDGEMENTS...

To my publisher Mathew Danswan for seeing the potential of this book and publishing it.

To Sheridan Voysey, the wonderful radio announcer who encouraged me to publish this book.

To Jayden & Caroline Lee; they have successfully completed my Daniel's Diet many times and can vouch for its positive outcome and they love it. Jayden and Caroline have a business called Bread Spot in Waukesha, Wisconsin, which sells natural food products.

To my many Pastor friends and all the Churches and community groups, for their support and feed-back on the diet.

To my daughter Nova and wife Kriste for helping with the book.

To my YWAM connection Sarah Seykora for her encouragement and support.

OTHER BOOKS BY PHILIP BRIDGEMAN

They can be purchased as paper back or EBooks from Philip's web site or online in Kindle format on Amazon.com

'Restoring Gods Natural Health Plan': A Biblical Perspective on Nutrition - for the Modern World.

'The Daniels's Way Recipe Guide' - A 10 Day Vegetarian Diet Plan. This is a specific recipe book for the 10 days while on; 'Daniel's Way to Weight Loss' (Daniel's Diet).

'Quick & Fast Meals – 7 Day Eating Plan for the Busy Women' - Easy and Fast Recipes, all under 15 minutes'. An EBook that is designed for the very busy and stressed woman (person). If this topic suits you then this book will give you a workable plan to follow.

'The 6 Week Low Carb Diet?' A Real Weight Loss Diet
This low carb diet plan is nearly the opposite of the Daniel's Diet. The effect of doing these two diets in tandem is very powerful and has wonderful results. You should lose 2kg a week and continue your journey to success. This diet plan is not long term and 6 weeks should be enough and then you can revisit Daniel's Way to Weight Loss again. Keep in mind you can reintroduce this 10 day plan at any time and as often as you want. You may continue for longer than the 10 days if you are wish.

Are You Tired, Lethargic & Can't Lose Weight? How you can Speed up your Metabolism & Regain your Energy - an eBook.

Daniel's Diet Lifestyle

The tremendous success of my first book, Daniel's Diet, has led me to write this second book as a continuation of the teaching about God's Natural Health Plan, answering more questions on health and covering topics like… What do I do after the 10 day Daniel's Diet?

A Testimony from Daniels Diet Lifestyle:

Hi Philip, What can I say….but….WOW!!

I thought your book, 'Daniel's Way to Weight Loss', was excellent, but your book Daniel's Diet Lifestyle is beyond that! The only word that comes to me is…..WOW!!! I could see God's anointing on your life with your first book, but this one has gone to a new level of excellence. Congratulations!

To put your knowledge down in written form, to get it in order of logic and in a simple form of understanding that even I can grasp, this is a big feat. God has given you many gifts and talents and you are putting them to good use…to bless me, others and all whom God leads to reading your books or brings in contact with you…you are such an encourager and an encouragement….thank you…**Jodie.**

Herbal Supplements (As Outlined in this Book)

Below are some effective vitamin combinations to assist you with Daniel's Diet.

Formula:
1. Weight Loss Support
2. Liver Detox Formula
3. Kidney and bowel detox formula
4. Adrenal Support (energy)
5. Beetroot, Carrot & Mixed Greens – Crystals/Powders.
6. FiberBlend™ (best herbal fibre mix that I know of)
7. Thyroid & Metabolism Support
8. Sugar Withdrawal Formula

9.   Non dairy- Protein Shakes
Would you like easy access to these formula's and products?

For quick ordering see Philip's website or email and quote the number listed above; www.wisdomforhealth.com philip@wisdomforhealth.net

Disclaimer –Herbal supplements mentioned in this book should not be used to diagnose, prevent, treat or cure any disease. The intention of this book is to outline the potential medicinal properties of certain herbs, but we are not liable for accuracy of these materials, for mistakes, errors, or omissions of any kind, nor for any loss or damage caused by a user's reliance on information obtained from this book. Any information contained on any of these pages is not intended to replace medical advice or treatment. Seek professional advice if you are on any medications, before using any herbs or diet changes.

Seminars for your Church!
As the founder of 'Wisdom for Health Ministries', we offer seminars and individual teaching (train the trainer) for anyone interested in learning under Philip and taking the teaching back to your church. As a presenter Philip encompasses both practical and spiritual subject matters, and is available to speak at business meetings, professional associations and church (all denominations). He regularly travels abroad communicating the message of health and wholeness. If you would like Philip to visit your church or group all you have to do is ask.

Philip's private naturopathic practice is located in Perth, Western Australia. Private consultations are available, both in person and for overseas and interstate people through long distance 'online consultation,' via Skype or phone

For further information and free downloads visit:
www.wisdomforheatlh.com
You can reach us on: **thebridgemanway@gmail.com**
Find us on Facebook: **www.facebook.com/restoringgodshealthplan/**

All the best with your Future Health & May God Bless You.
Philip Bridgeman